THE HEALTH COOKBOOK

Lower Your Blood Pressure in a Few Weeks
Thanks to These DASH Life-Changing
Recipes

Dash and Delicious

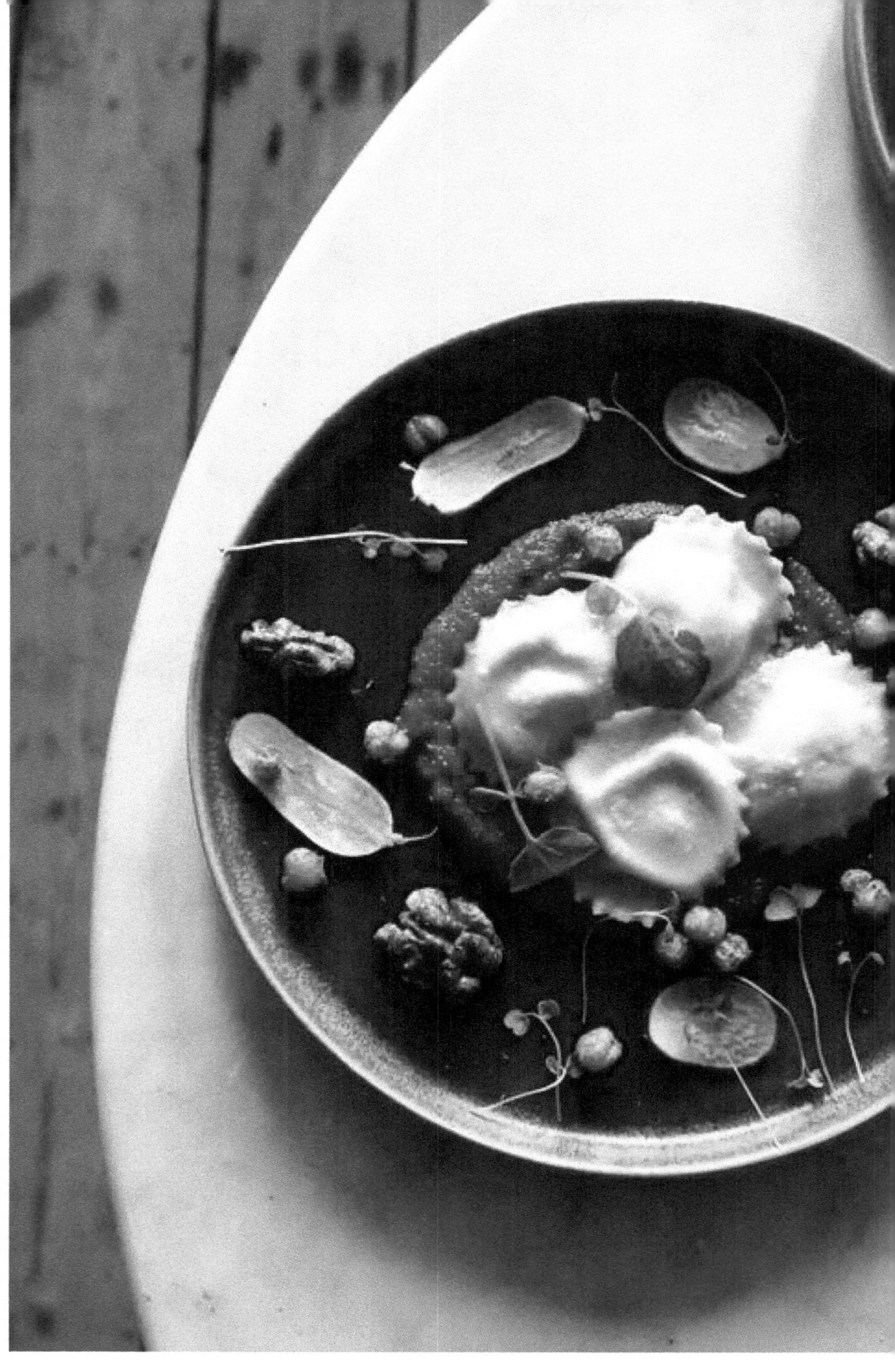

the reader will render any resulting actions solely under their purview. There are no scenarios in which the publisher or the original author of this work can be in any fashion deemed liable for any hardship or damages that may befall them after undertaking the information described herein.

Additionally, the information in the following pages is intended only for informational purposes and should thus be thought of as universal. As befitting its nature, it is presented without assurance regarding its prolonged validity or interim quality. Trademarks that are mentioned are done without written consent and can in no way be considered an endorsement from the trademark holder.

Table of Contents

INTRODUCTION

The last two decades have witnessed a doubling in the number of people with high blood pressure, many of whom are not good at controlling their symptoms. Our millennial lifestyle has played a great role in producing this worrisome result.

To counter this, scientists introduced the DASH diet, which is an effective way to counteract hypertension among people. The diet is results of careful study of the various food items that will help people control their blood pressure levels.

What is the DASH diet?

Endorsed by the United States National Heart, Lung, and Blood Institute, the DASH (Dietary Approaches to Stop Hypertension) diet studies the nutrient composition of food to prepare unique dietary strategies to eliminate the foods that contribute to high blood pressure.

The United States Department of Health and Human Services began to look for ways to deal with hypertension and eliminate the various risks that are associated with it. Researchers found that people who consume more vegetables or followed a plant-based diet had less of a risk of high blood pressure. This, therefore, became the foundation of the DASH diet.

This diet focuses on foods that are non-processed and more organic. Whole grains, fruits, vegetables, and lean meats form the essential components. In extreme cases, where signs of heart-related ailments due to high blood pressure are present, it is advised for the patient to go vegan for some time to lower issues related to hypertension.

The Dash diet strict dietary sodium because too much salt and oil significantly raise blood pressure. The dietary guidelines of the DASH diet significantly reduce the intake of salt. The recipes in the DASH diet are a wholesome mix of green vegetables, natural fruits, low-fat dairy foods, and lean protein such as chicken, fish, and beans. Besides limiting the intake of salt, the rule of thumb is to minimize food items rich in red meat, processed sugars, and composite fat.

Benefits of the DASH diet

The benefits of the DASH diet go beyond reducing hypertension and heart ailments.

- **Controlling blood pressure**

The force exerted on our blood vessels and organs when the blood passes through them is a measure of blood pressure in the human body. When blood pressure increases beyond a certain level, it can lead to various bodily malfunctions, including heart failure.

Blood pressure is counted in two numbers: systolic pressure and diastolic pressure. Normal blood systolic pressure in adults is below 120 mmHg, while the diastolic pressure is typically below 80 mmHg. Anyone over these limits is said to be suffering from high blood pressure.

The restriction of sodium intake and reliance on vegetables, healthy fat, lean meat, and fruits in the DASH diet greatly controls blood pressure. Effective use of the DASH diet can control the systolic blood pressure by an average change of 12 mmHg and can control the diastolic blood pressure by 5 mmHg.

The DASH diet is not reserved for people suffering from hypertension; it can also work well for people with normal blood pressure. The trick is to consume normal amounts of salt along with the dietary recommendations given in the DASH diet.

- **Weight loss**

People with high blood pressure are advised to maintain an optimal weight, as extra weight may translate into health complications. Obesity along with high blood pressure can lead to heart and organ failure. With the help of the DASH diet, one can lower their blood pressure while also reducing their weight. The credit for this goes to the healthy foods recommended in the DASH diet.

Further, the DASH diet has shown signs of other health benefits:

- **Lowers the risk of cancer**

People on the DASH diets have a lower risk of colorectal and breast cancers.

- **Checks metabolic syndrome**

The diet reduces the risk of metabolic syndrome.

- **Controls diabetes**

The diet is very beneficial for people with type 2 diabetes.

- **Heart diseases**

The diet reduces the risk of heart disease and stroke.

DASH Food Guidelines - What to Eat and Avoid on the Dash Diet

On the DASH diet, excessive fats, salt, and spices need to be avoided. Cut all empty carbohydrates from the diet completely, opting for food that is rich in vitamins, protein, and fiber.

DASH Foods and Serving Sizes

One of the important features of the DASH diet is 'proportion.' Correct proportion of food portions is essential. How do you determine the proportions? Based on extensive research and years of studies, experts have recommendations for serving sizes and combination, depending on nutritional value. The following table shows the serving size of all the major categories of food in a certain caloric diet.

Foods to Enjoy

On a broader scale, this diet plan doesn't restrict the use of most food items, but it does limit their amount. Following is the list of items that can be taken on the DASH Diet:

Seeds	Fruits	Poultry
Nuts	Vegetables	Seafood
Grains	low fat or no-fat dairy products	Beef
		Pork

- **Vegetables: 4-5 Servings Daily**

A half cup of cooked or raw vegetables or 1 cup of leafy vegetables constitutes one serving on the DASH diet. Carrots, greens, sweet potatoes, broccoli, and tomatoes can all be included by adjusting the values of the serving. Set the limiting values and fill in as many vegetables as you can.

- **Grains: 6-8 Servings Daily**

Rice, pasta, cereal, quinoa, bread, etc., are all considered grains. A single serving means 1 oz. of cereal, 1 slice of bread, or a half cup of pasta or rice. Keeping these proportions in mind, you can consume a single serving six to eight times per day. How you divide these servings in a day depends completely on you. Whole grains are recommended most as they are rich in fiber. Similarly, go for brown rice and whole-wheat pasta; both have more fiber.

- **Dairy: 2 - 3 Servings Daily**

Dairy products include cheese, milk, and yogurt. All are a source of protein, calcium, and vitamin D. As long as the dairy products are free from saturated fats or contain a low amount of fat, they are good to go for the DASH diet. A single serving means 1 cup of low-fat yogurt or skim milk or 1.5 oz. of part-skim cheese.

- **Fats and oils: 2 - 3 servings Daily**

Good cholesterol fats and plant-based fats are great for the body; in fact, they strengthen the immune system and aid the absorption of vitamins in the body. Excluding them completely from your diet is unnecessary and unhealthy. Place them in the middle category, having three servings a day, and focus more on mono-saturated fats.

- **Fruits: 4 - 5 Servings Daily**

One medium-sized fresh fruit or canned fruits make a single serving. Fruits are packed with fiber, minerals, and vitamins, so they are good additions to the DASH diet. They generally have low or zero sodium. Four oz. of fruit juice makes up a single serving. Add all the varieties to set the final figures up to five servings in a day.

- **Sweets: 5 servings a week**

Sweets should be consumed least. Five servings a week is more than enough. One serving is one tbsp sugar, a half cup of sorbet, or a cup of lemonade. A moderate use of sweets is necessary; complete deprivation would result in more harm.

- **Seeds, Nuts, and legumes: 4 - 5 Servings Per Week**

This category includes lentils, kidney beans, and peas, edibles seeds like sunflower, sesame, and almonds. They all are a great source of potassium, protein, and magnesium. They are rich in fiber and antioxidants, which prevent cancer and cardiovascular diseases.

Foods to Avoid

Food that can cause hypertension, high blood pressure, high blood sugar levels, and obesity are all forbidden on a DASH diet. The following list of items should be limited:

1. Salt
2. Sugary beverages
3. Processed food
4. High fat dairy products
5. Salted nuts
6. Excessive animal-based fats

Some Questions regarding the DASH DIET

Q. Can people without hypertension also use the DASH diet?

The DASH diet was indeed created to reduce the risk of hypertension and control blood pressure, but owing to its wide-ranging health benefits, anyone can use this diet for better health.

Q. How long should a dieter stick to the DASH diet to see the results?

It is best to make this plan a lifestyle if you are a hypertension patient, rather than adopting it for a few days or months. Since it does not harm you in the long run, it is up to you and your health expert to follow this diet plan as long as needed.

Q. What can you drink on the DASH diet?

All low-calorie, sodium-free, and sugar-free drinks are most suitable for the DASH diet, which make water a perfect candidate. However, sugar-free juices and drinks are also a good option.

Q. Can you use the DASH diet when you are taking medications for hypertension or high blood pressure?

It is not suggested to use the DASH diet when you are on any medication as there can be interactions. Ask for your doctor's opinion on this matter and take his advice to continue the medications along with the diet or not.

BREAKFAST

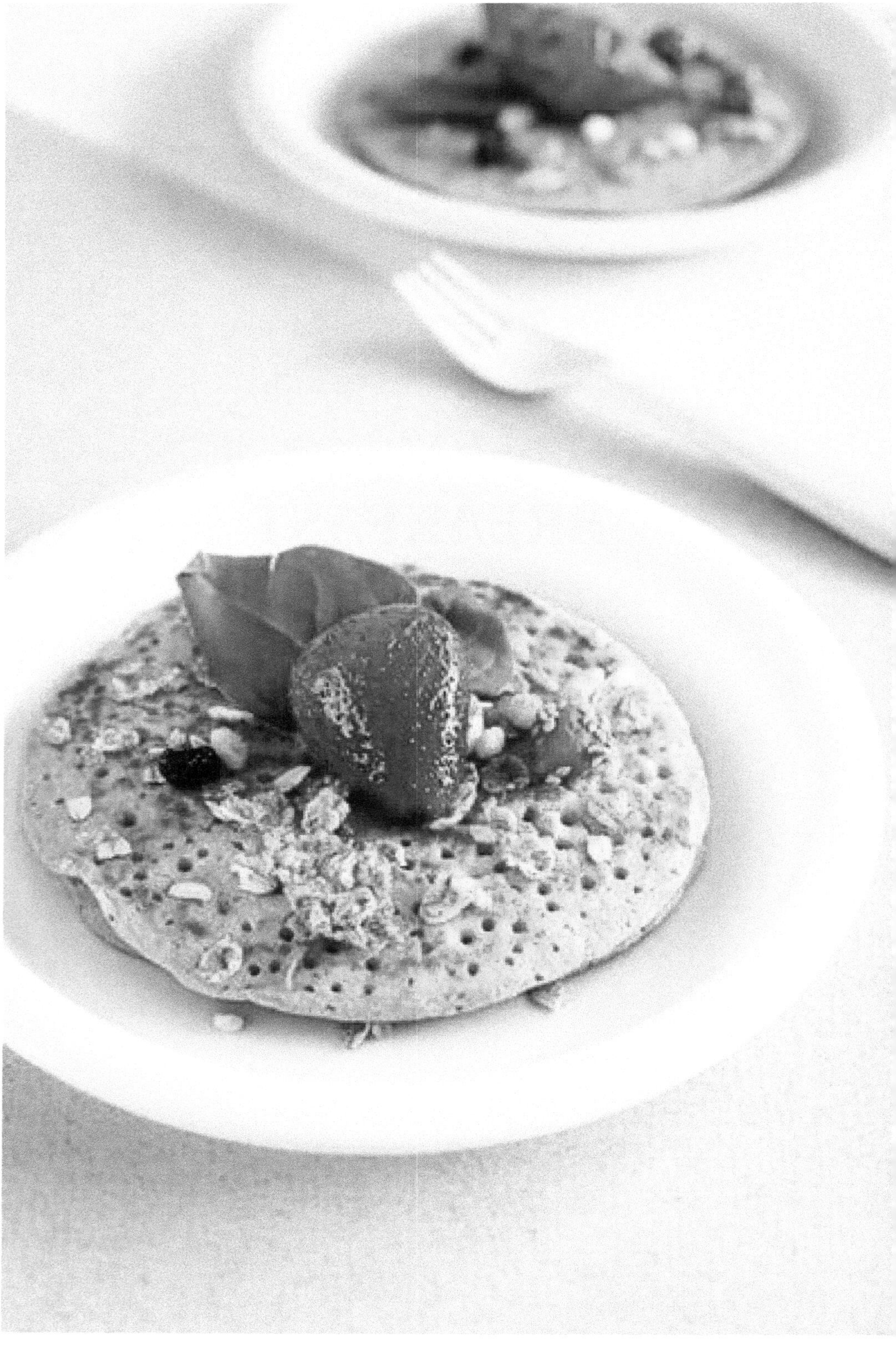

8 Servings

Preparation Time: 30 minutes

Ingredients

- ¾ cup Coconut cream
- 2 cups Coconut milk
- 1 cup Brown rice
- 2 tablespoons Coconut sugar
- 1 teaspoon Vanilla extract

Directions

- In a pot, combine the milk with the rice and the other ingredients, stir, bring to a simmer and cook over medium heat for 20 minutes.
- Stir the mix again, divide into bowls and serve for breakfast.

Vanilla Rice and Cherries

6 Servings

Preparation Time: 35 minutes

Ingredients

- 2 cups Coconut milk
- ½ teaspoon Vanilla extract
- 1 tablespoon Coconut, shredded
- 2 tablespoons Coconut sugar
- 1 cup Brown rice
- ¼ cup Cherries, pitted and halved
- Cooking spray

Directions

- Put the milk in a pot, add the sugar and the coconut, stir and bring to a simmer over medium heat.
- Add the rice and the other ingredients, simmer for 25 minutes stirring often, divide into bowls and serve.

Rice Bowls

6 Servings

Preparation Time: 35 minutes

Ingredients

- 3 tablespoons Coconut sugar
- 1 cup Brown rice
- 2 cups Almond milk
- 1 tablespoon Ginger, grated
- 1 teaspoon Cinnamon powder

Directions

- Put the milk in a pot, bring to a simmer over medium heat, add the rice and the other ingredients, stir, cook for 25 minutes, divide into bowls and serve.

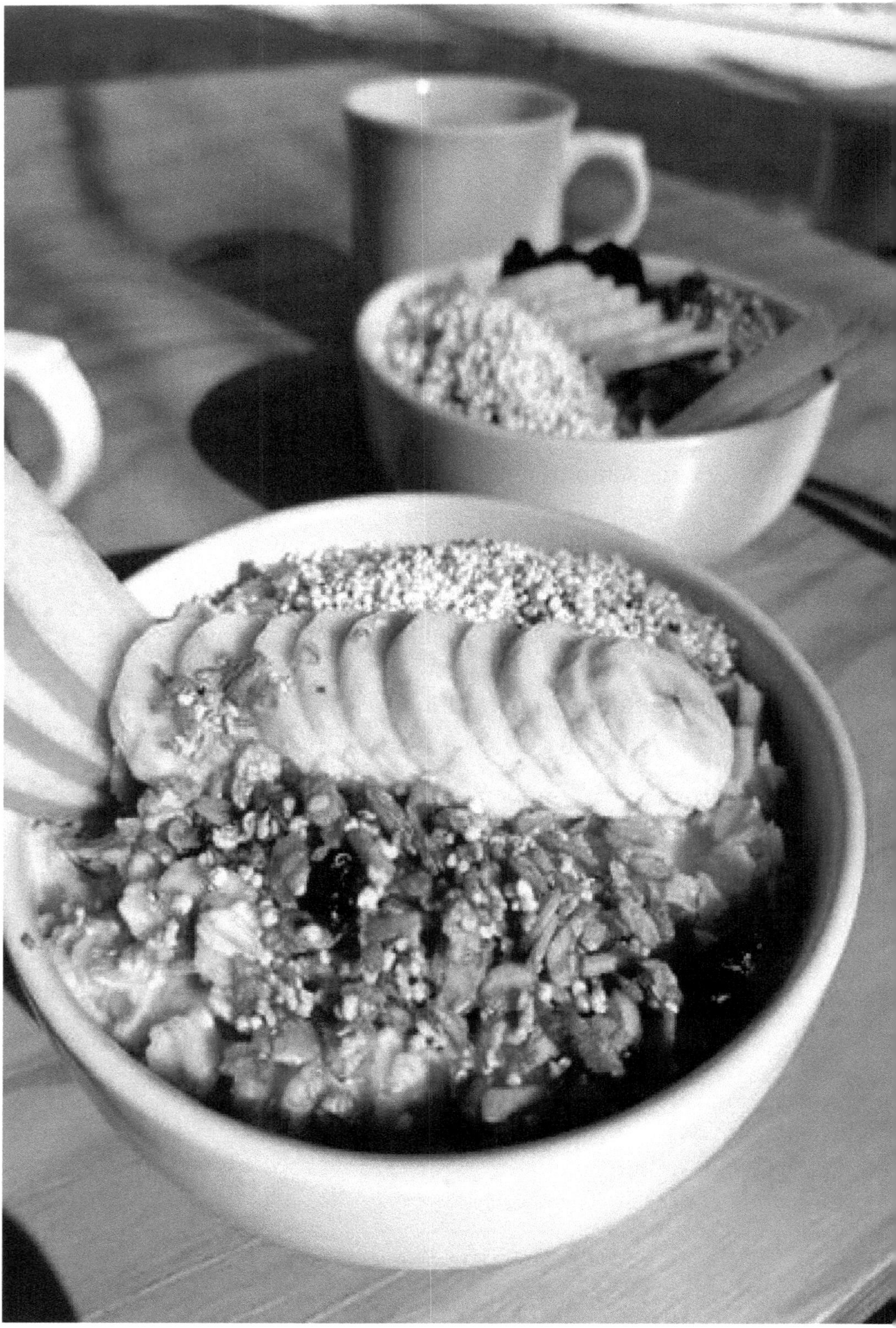

Hash Browns Casserole

6 Servings

Preparation Time: 45 minutes

Ingredients

- 1 tablespoon Olive oil
- 6 ounces low-sodium Sausage, chopped
- 1 pound Hash browns
- 6 Eggs, whisked
- 1 Red onion, chopped
- 1 Chili pepper, chopped
- ¼ teaspoon Chili powder
- A pinch of Black pepper

Directions

- Heat up a pan with the oil over medium heat, add the onion and the sausage, stir and brown for 5 minutes.
- Add the hash browns and the other ingredients except the eggs and pepper, stir and cook for 5 minutes more.
- Pour the eggs mixed with the black pepper over the sausage mix, introduce the pan in the oven and bake at 370 degrees F for 25 minutes.
- Divide the mix between plates and serve for breakfast,

Mushroom and Rice Mix

6 Servings

Preparation Time: 40 minutes

Ingredient

- 2 cups low-sodium Chicken stock
- 1 tablespoon Cilantro, chopped
- 1 red Onion, chopped
- 1 cup Brown rice
- 2 Garlic cloves, minced
- 2 tablespoons Olive oil
- ½ cup fat-free Cheddar cheese, grated
- ½ pound white Mushroom, sliced
- Black pepper to the taste

Directions

- Heat up a pan with the oil over medium heat, add the onion, garlic and mushrooms, stir and cook for 5-6 minutes.
- Add the rice and the rest of the ingredients, bring to a simmer and cook over medium heat for 25 minutes stirring often.
- Divide the rice, mix between bowls and serve for breakfast.

Tomato Eggs

6 Servings

Preparation Time: 30 minutes

Ingredients

- 1 yellow Onion, chopped
- 1 tablespoon Olive oil
- ½ cup low-fat Milk
- Black pepper to the taste
- 8 Eggs, whisked
- 1 cup Baby spinach, chopped
- 1 cup Cherry tomatoes, cubed
- ¼ cup fat-free Cheddar, grated

Directions

- Heat up a pan with the oil over medium heat, add the onion, stir and cook for 2-3 minutes.
- Add the spinach and tomatoes, stir and cook for 2 minutes more.
- Add the eggs mixed with the milk and black pepper and toss gently.
- Sprinkle the cheddar on top, introduce the pan in the oven and cook at 390 degrees F for 15 minutes.
- Divide between plates and serve.

Zucchini Almond Oatmeal

6 Servings

Preparation Time: 25 minutes

Ingredients

- 2 teaspoons Cinnamon powder
- 1 cup steel cut Oats
- 3 cups Almond milk
- 1 tablespoon fat-free Butter
- 1 teaspoon Pumpkin pie spice
- 1 cup Zucchinis, grated

Directions

- Heat up a pan with the milk over medium heat, add the oats and the other ingredients, toss, bring to a simmer and cook for 20 minutes, stirring from time to time.
- Divide the oatmeal into bowls and serve for breakfast.

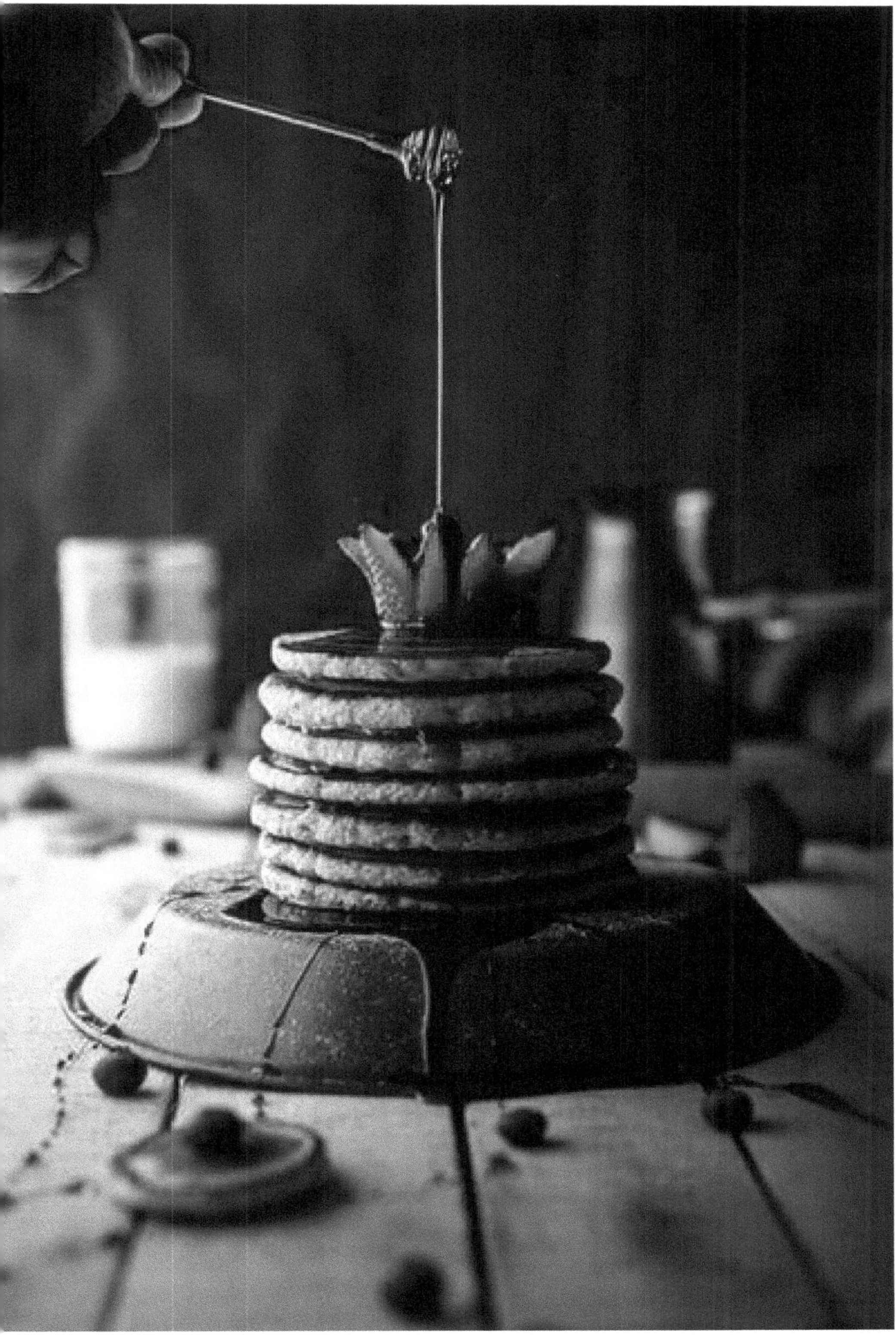

6 Servings

Preparation Time: 25 minutes

Ingredients

- 1 cup Raisins
- 1 cup Almonds
- 2 cups Coconut milk
- 1 cup Coconut, shredded
- ½ cup Maple syrup
- ½ teaspoon Vanilla extract

Directions

- Put the milk in a pot, bring to a simmer over medium heat, add the coconut and the other ingredients, and cook for 20 minutes, stirring from time to time.
- Divide the mix into bowls and serve warm for breakfast.

JUICES & SMOOTHIES

Apple & Pomegranate Juice

2 Servings

Preparation Time: 10 minutes

Ingredients

- 1½ C. fresh Pomegranate seeds
- 2 tsps fresh Lemon juice
- 2 large Apples, cored and sliced
- Pinch of Ground Black pepper

Directions

- In a food processor, add all ingredients and extract the juice according to the manufacturer's directions.
- Transfer into 2 glasses and serve immediately.

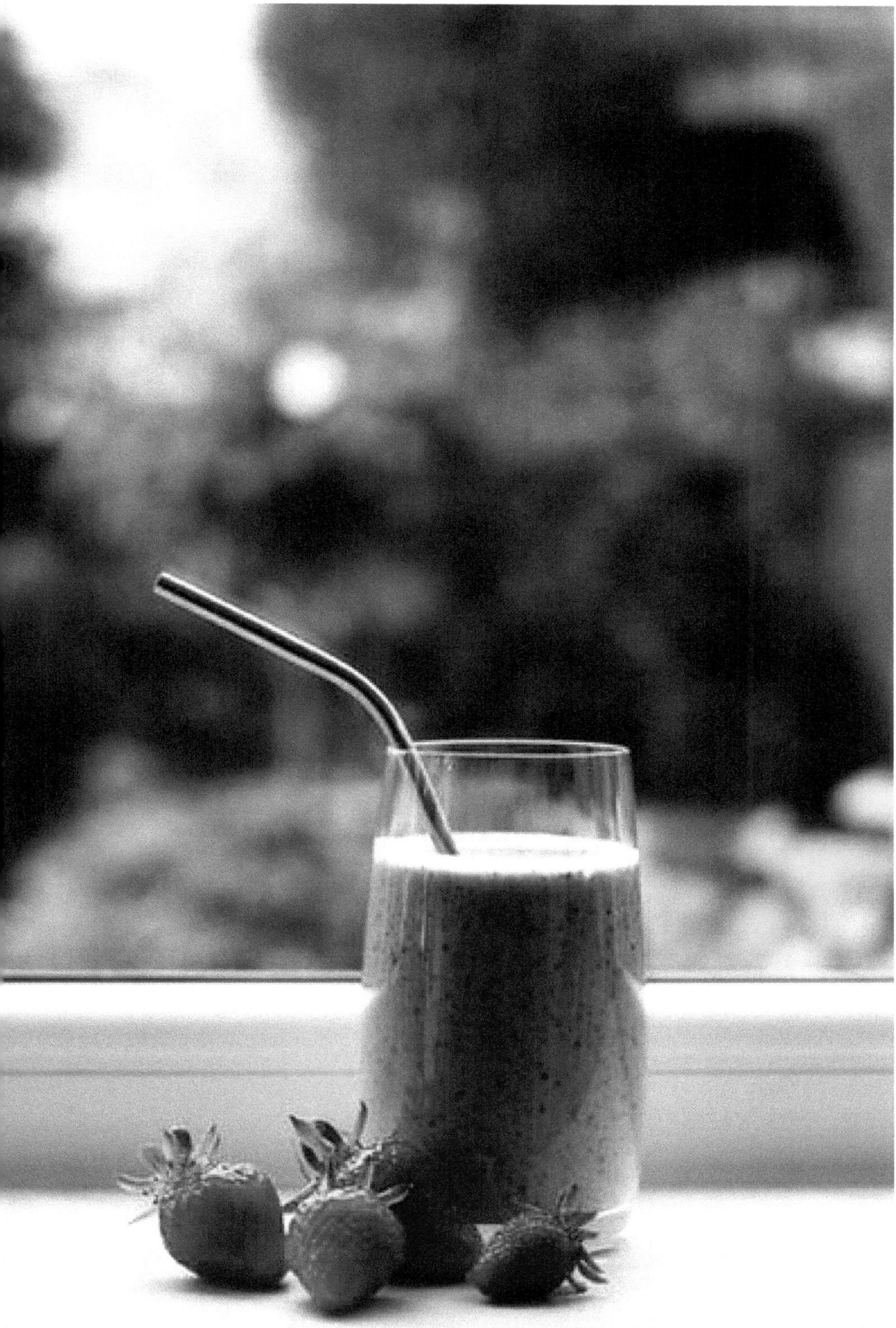

Apple, Grapefruit & Carrot Juice

3 Servings

Preparation Time: 12 minutes

Ingredients

- 2 large Apples, cored and sliced
- 3 medium Carrots, peeled and chopped
- 2 medium Grapefruits, peeled and seeded
- 1 tsp fresh Lemon juice

Directions

- In a food processor, add all ingredients and extract the juice according to the manufacturer's directions.
- Transfer into 3 glasses and serve immediately.

Apple & Spinach Juice

4 Servings

Preparation Time: 15 minutes

Ingredients

- 4 large green Apples, cored and sliced
- ¼ C. fresh Parsley leaves
- 2 Lemon, peeled and seeded
- 8 C. fresh Spinach leaves
- 2 tbsps fresh Ginger, peeled
- 2 C. chilled filtered Water

Directions

- In a blender, add all ingredients and pulse well.
- Through a strainer, strain the juice and transfer into 4 glasses. Serve immediately.

Pumpkin Smoothie

4 Servings

Preparation Time: 12 minutes

Ingredients

- 1 C. homemade Pumpkin puree
- 1 tsp ground Flaxseeds
- 1½ C. unsweetened Almond Milk
- 1 medium Banana, peeled and sliced
- ¼ tsp ground Cinnamon
- ¼ C. Ice cubes

Directions

- In a high-speed blender, add all ingredients and pulse until smooth.
- Transfer into 4 serving glasses and serve immediately.

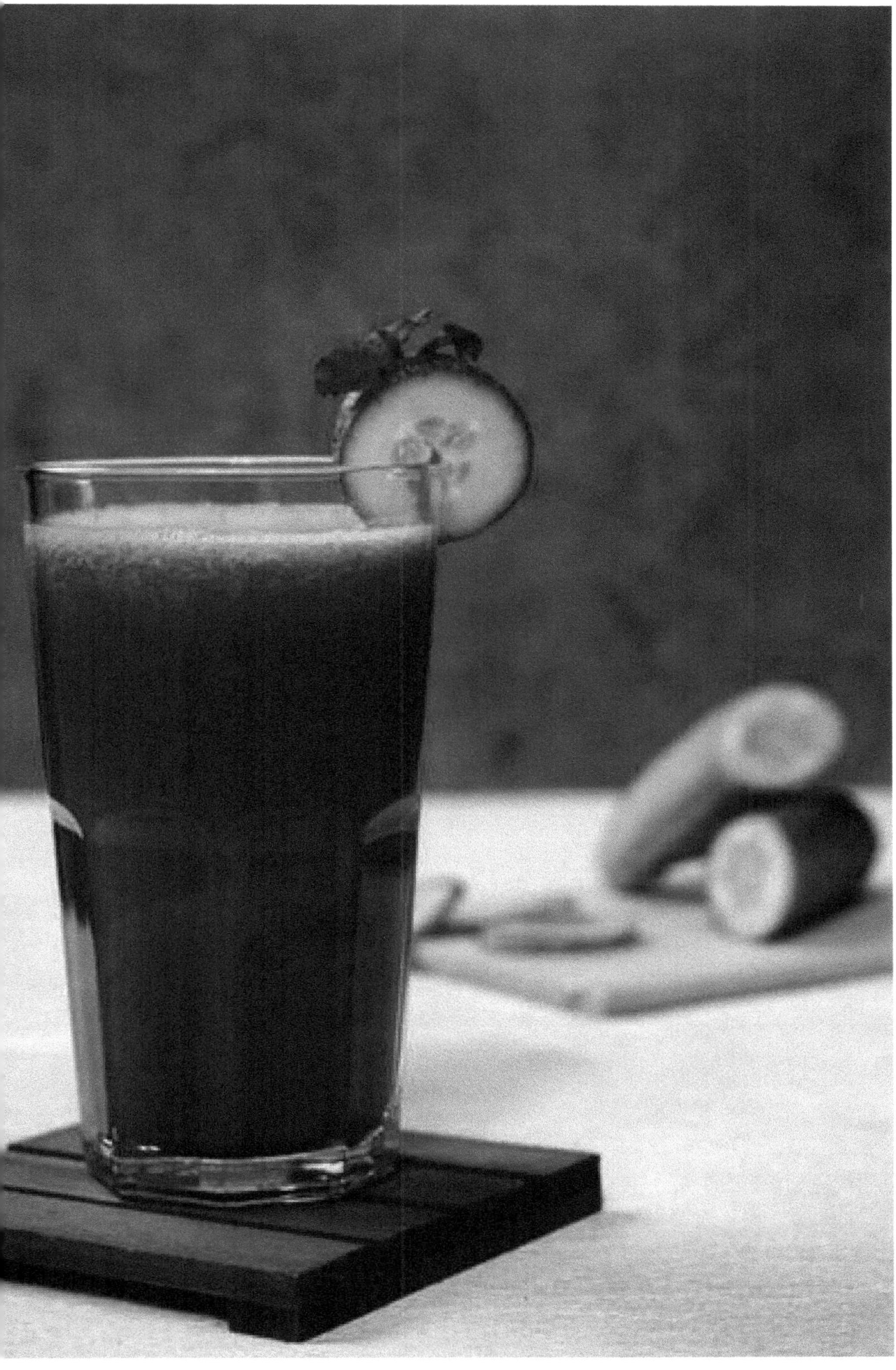

Cucumber& Greens Smoothie

2 Servings

Preparation Time: 12 minutes

Ingredients

- 1 small Cucumber, peeled and chopped
- ½ C. Lettuce, torn
- ¼ C. fresh Mint leaves
- 1 tsp fresh Lemon juice
- ¼ C. Ice cubes
- 2 C. mixed fresh Greens
- ¼ C. fresh Parsley leaves
- 2-3 drops liquid Stevia
- 1½ C. filtered Water

Directions

- In a high-speed blender, add all ingredients and pulse until smooth.
- Transfer into 2 serving glasses and serve immediately.

Chocolaty Avocado Smoothie

3 Servings

Preparation Time: 15 minutes

Ingredients

- 1 medium Avocado, peeled, pitted and chopped
- ½ tsp Organic Vanilla extract
- ¼ C. Ice cubes
- 1 small Banana, peeled and sliced
- 3 tbsps Cacao powder
- 1¾ C. chilled fat-free Milk

Directions

- In a high-speed blender, add all ingredients and pulse until smooth.
- Transfer into 3 serving glasses and serve immediately.

Avocado & Spinach Smoothie

2 Servings

Preparation Time: 12 minutes

Ingredients

- 2 C. fresh baby Spinach
- 1 tbsp Hemp seeds
- 3-4 drops liquid Stevia
- ½ of Avocado, peeled, pitted and chopped
- ½ tsp ground Cinnamon
- 2 C. chilled filtered Water

Directions

- In a high-speed blender, add all ingredients and pulse until smooth.
- Transfer into 2 serving glasses and serve immediately.

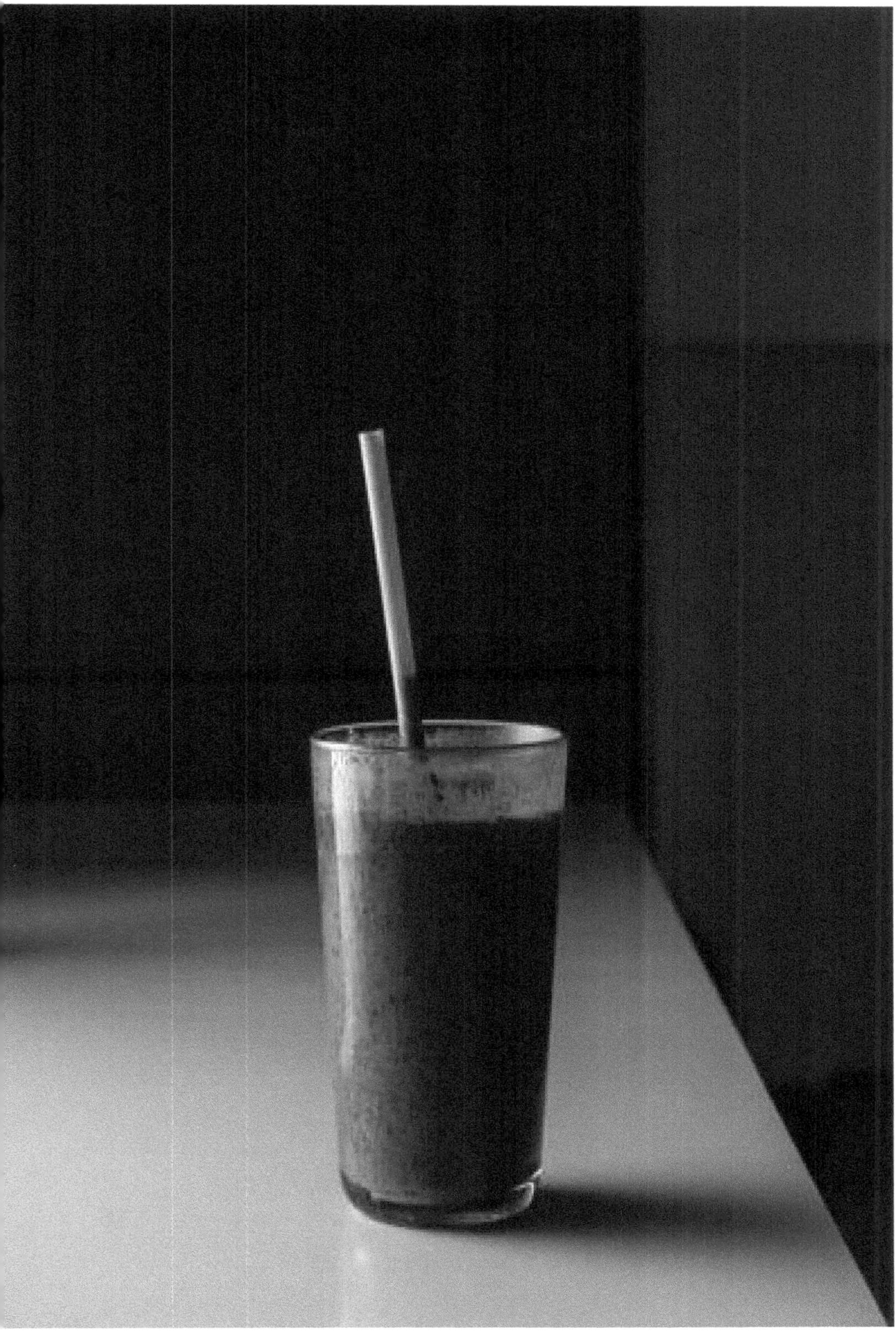

Green Veggie Smoothie

3 Servings

Preparation Time: 10 minutes

Ingredients

- 1 C. fresh Spinach
- ½ of small Green bell pepper, seeded and chopped
- 2 C. chilled filtered Water
- ¼ C. Broccoli Florets, chopped
- ¼ C. green Cabbage, chopped
- 3-4 drops liquid Stevia

Directions

- In a high-speed blender, add all ingredients and pulse until smooth.
- Transfer into 3 serving glasses and serve immediately.

LUNCH

Shrimp & Tomato Casserole

6 servings

Preparation Time: 45 minutes

Ingredients

- ¼ C. Olive Oil
- 1½ lbs. large shrimp, peeled and deveined
- ¼ tsp red pepper flakes, crushed
- ¾ C. low-sodium chicken broth
- 4 oz. feta cheese, crumbled
- 1 tbsp Garlic, minced
- ¾ tsp dried oregano, crushed
- ¼ C. fresh parsley, chopped
- 2¼ C. tomatoes, chopped

Directions

- Preheat the oven to 350 °F. In a large pan, heat the oil over medium-high heat and sauté the Garlic for about 1 minute.
- Add the shrimp, oregano and red pepper flakes and cook for about 4-5 minutes. Stir in the parsley and Pinch of salt immediately transfer into a casserole dish evenly.

38

- In the same pan, add broth over medium heat and simmer for about 2-3 minutes. Stir in tomatoes and cook for about 2-3 minutes. Pour the tomato mixture over shrimp mixture evenly.
- Top with cheese evenly. Bake for about 15-20 minutes or until top becomes golden brown.

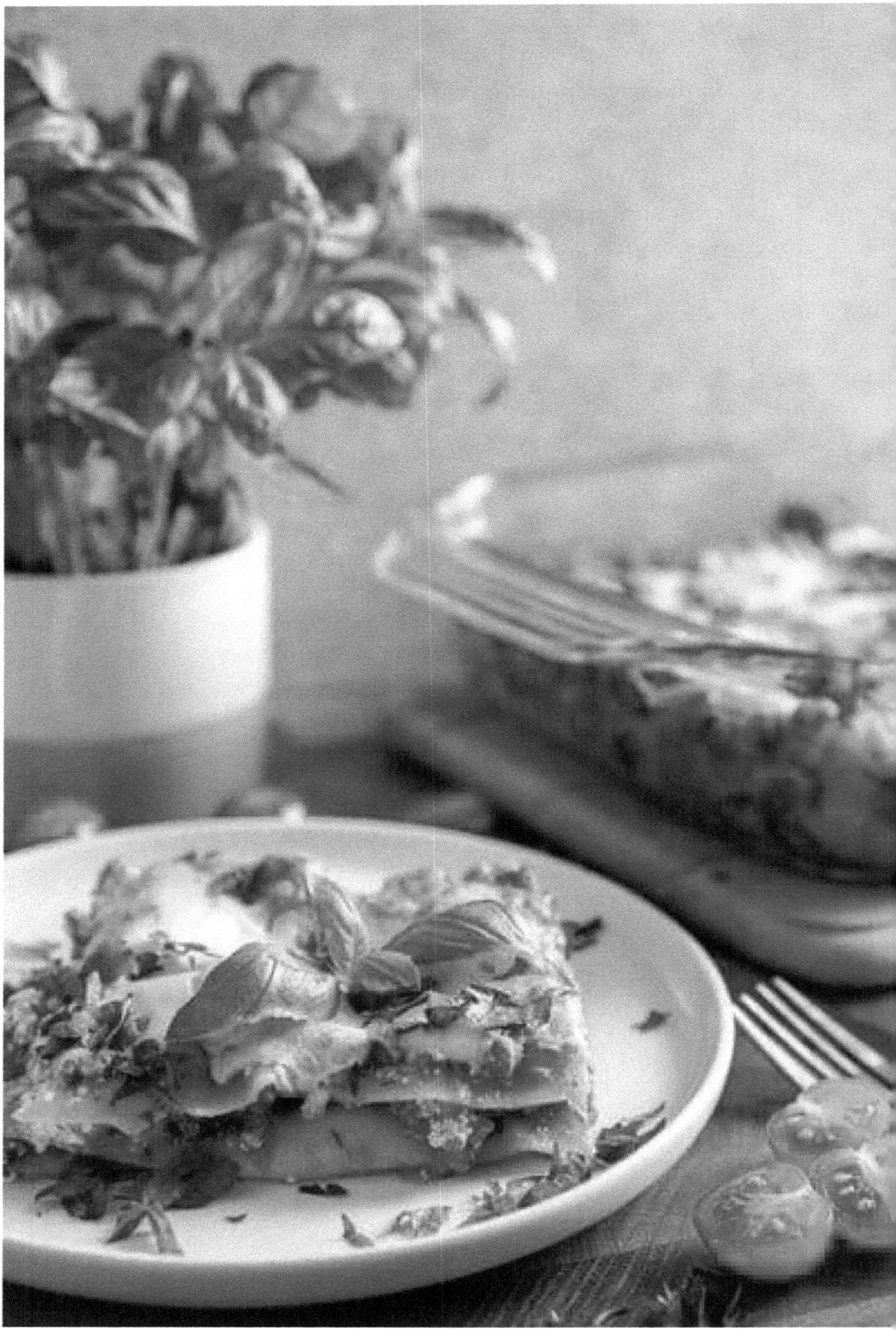

Prawns & Veggie Curry

6 servings

Preparation Time: 20 minutes

Ingredients

- 2 tbsps Olive Oil
- 1 tbsp fresh Ginger, chopped finely
- 2½ tsps curry powder
- 2 medium bell peppers, seeded and sliced
- 1 C. low-fat sour cream
- Freshly ground Black pepper, to taste
- 1 medium Onion, sliced
- 3 Garlic cloves, chopped finely
- 3 medium carrots, peeled and sliced thinly
- 1½ lbs. prawns, peeled and deveined
- ¼ C. water
- 3 tbsps fresh basil leaves, chopped

Directions

- In a large pan, heat the oil over medium-high heat and sauté Onion for about 4-5 minutes.
- Add Ginger, Garlic and curry powder and sauté for about 1 minute. Add bell peppers and carrot and sauté for about 3-4 minutes.

- Add prawns, sour cream and water and stir to combine.
- Cook for about 3-4 minutes, stirring, occasionally.
- Stir in Black pepper and remove from heat. Serve hot with the garnishing of basil.

Beef Burger

8 Servings

Preparation Time: 25 minutes

Ingredients

- 1 lb. lean ground Beef
- 1 medium beet, trimmed, peeled and chopped finely
- 2 Serrano peppers, seeded and chopped finely
- Freshly ground Black pepper, to taste
- 8 C. fresh baby kale
- 1 carrot, peeled and chopped finely
- 1 small Onion, chopped finely
- 1 tbsp fresh Cilantro, chopped finely
- Pinch of salt
- 3 tbsps Olive Oil

Directions

- For burgers in a large bowl, add all ingredients except oil and mix until well combined.
- Make 12 equal-sized patties from mixture. In a large non-stick pan, heat oil over medium heat. Add patties in 3 batches and cook for about 3-4 minutes per side or until golden brown. Divide kale in serving plates evenly.
- Place 2 burgers onto each plate and serve.

Stuffed leg of lamb

8 Servings

Preparation Time: 1 hour 40 minutes

Ingredients

- 1/3 C. fresh parsley, minced
- 3 tbsps Olive Oil, divided
- 1 (4-lb.) boneless leg of lamb, butter flied and trimmed
- ½ C. Kalamata olives, pitted and chopped
- 1 tsp fresh lemon zest, finely grated
- 8 Garlic cloves, minced and divided
- Freshly ground Black pepper, to taste
- 1/3 C. yellow Onion, minced
- 1 bunch fresh kale, trimmed and chopped
- ½ C. feta cheese, crumbled
-

Directions

- In a large baking dish, add the parsley, 4 Garlic cloves, 2 tbsps of oil, salt, and Black pepper and mix until well combined.
- Add the leg of lamb and generously coat with parsley mixture. Set aside at room temperature.

- In a large pan, heat the remaining oil over medium heat and sauté the Onion and remaining Garlic for about 4-5 minutes.
- Add the kale and cook for about 4-5 minutes.
- Remove from the heat and set aside to cool for at least 10 minutes.
- Stir in the remaining ingredients. Preheat the oven to 450 ºF.
- Grease a shallow roasting pan. Place the leg of lamb onto a smooth surface, cut-side up.
- Place kale mixture in the center, leaving 1-inch border from both sides.
- Roll the short side to seal the stuffing and with a kitchen string, tightly tie the roll at many places.
- Arrange the roll into prepared roasting pan, seam-side down.
- Roast for about 15 minutes. Now, adjust the temperature of oven to 350 ºF. Roast for about 1-1¼ hours.
- Remove the leg of lamb from oven and place onto a cutting board for about 10-20 minutes before slicing.
- With a sharp knife, cut the roll into desired size slices and serve.

Baked Lamb with Cauliflower

8 Servings

Preparation Time: 24 hours

Ingredients

- 2 tbsps Olive Oil
- 1 Onion, chopped
- 1 tsp ground cumin
- Freshly ground Black pepper, to taste
- 1 medium head cauliflower, cut into 1-inch florets
- 3 lbs. lamb stew meat, trimmed and cubed
- 2 Garlic cloves, minced
- ½ tsp cayenne pepper
- 2¼ C. low-sodium chicken broth
- 2 C. tomatoes, chopped finely

Directions

- Preheat the oven to 300 °F.
- In a small bowl, mix together spices and set aside. In a large oven-proof pan, heat oil over medium heat.
- Add lamb and cook for about 10 minutes or until browned from all sides.
- Transfer the lamb into a bowl.

- In the same pan, add Onion and sauté for about 3-4 minutes. Add Garlic and spice mixture and sauté for about 1 minute.
- Add cooked lamb, broth and tomatoes and bring to a gentle boil.
- Immediately, cover the pan and transfer into oven.
- Bake for about 1½ hours.
- Remove from oven and stir in cauliflower.
- Bake for about 30 minute more or until cauliflower is done completely.

Chicken with broccoli & mushrooms

6 servings

Preparation Time: 40 minutes

Ingredients

- 3 tbsps Olive Oil
- 1 medium Onion, chopped
- 16 oz. small broccoli florets
- Pinch of salt
- 1 lb. skinless, boneless chicken breast, cubed
- 6 Garlic cloves, minced
- ¼ C. water
- Freshly ground Black pepper, to taste

Directions

- Heat the oil in a large pan over medium heat and cook the chicken cubes for about 4-5 minutes.

- With a slotted spoon, transfer the chicken cubes onto a plate.

- In the same pan, add the Onion and sauté for about 4-5 minutes.

- Add the mushrooms and cook for about 4-5 minutes.

- Stir in the cooked chicken, broccoli and water and cook, covered for about 8-10 minutes, stirring occasionally.

- Stir in salt and Black pepper and remove from heat.

- Serve hot.

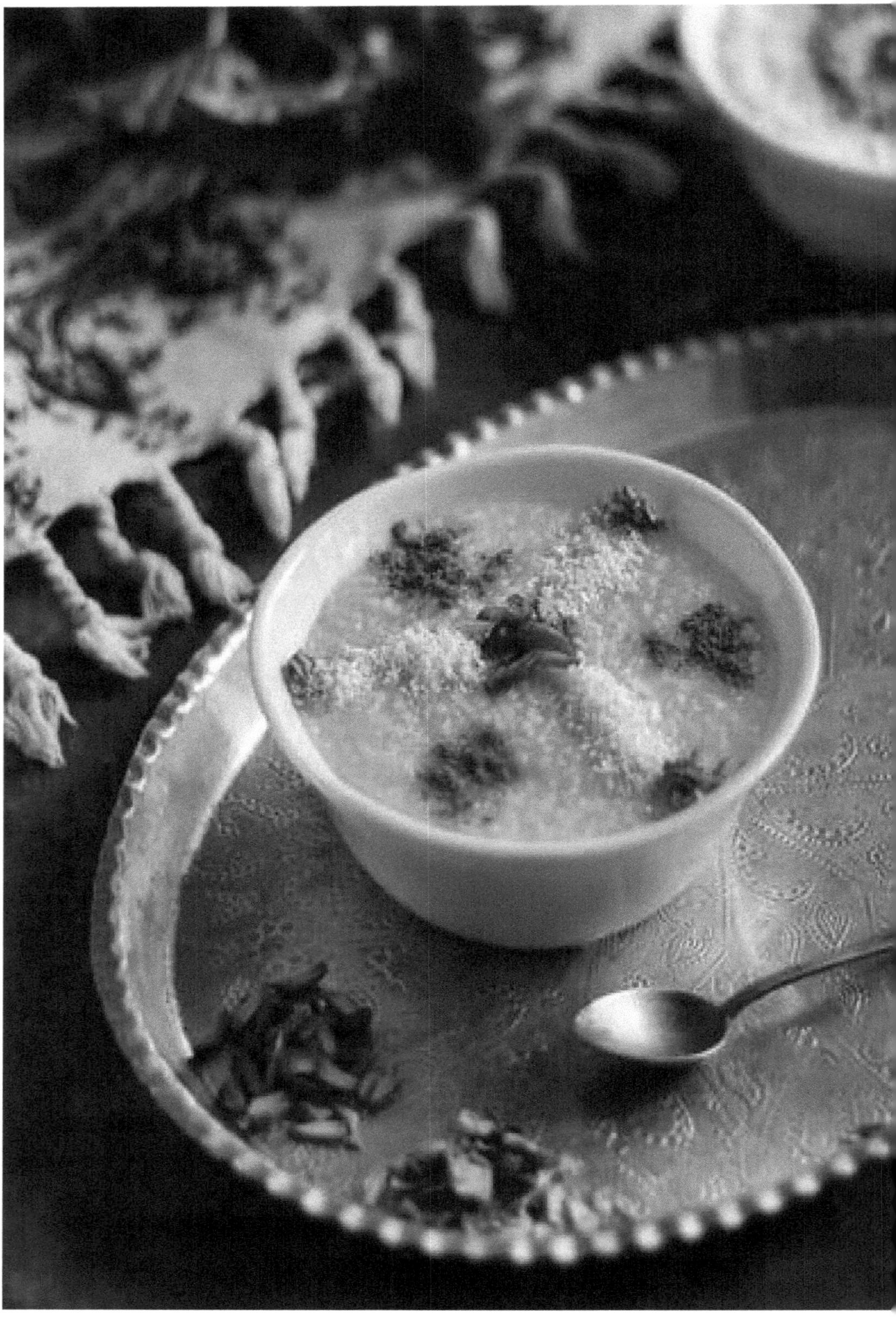

Chicken with olives & tomatoes

4 Servings

Preparation Time: 25 minutes

Ingredients

- 4 (5-oz.) boneless, skinless chicken breasts, trimmed
- 2-3 tbsps fresh oregano, chopped
- 1 C. cherry tomatoes, quartered
- ½ C. feta cheese, crumbled
- ½ C. plus 1 tbsp Olive Oil, divided
- ½ C. fresh lemon juice
- 1 tsp Garlic, chopped finely
- 1/3 C. Kalamata olives, pitted and sliced
- Freshly ground Black pepper, to taste

Directions

- With a knife, make small diagonal cuts on the top of each chicken breast. In a bowl, add ½ C. of the oil, lemon juice, oregano and Garlic and mix well. Transfer about ¼ C. of the oil mixture in another bowl and reserve it.
- In a Ziploc bag, add the chicken breasts and remaining oil mixture. Seal the bag and shake to coat well. Refrigerate to marinate for at least 1 hour.

- Remove from the refrigerator and place the chicken aside until it comes to room temperature. In the bowl of the reserved marinade, add the tomatoes, olives and feta cheese and gently stir to combine.
- In a large heavy-bottomed pan, heat about the remaining oil over medium-high heat and cook the chicken breasts for about 3-5 minutes per side. Stir in the Black pepper and remove from the heat. Transfer the chicken breasts onto serving plates and serve with the topping of feta mixture.

Chicken & Beans Chili

6 servings

Preparation Time: 45 minutes

Ingredients

- 2 tbsps Olive Oil
- 1 C. Onion, chopped
- 1½ tsps dried Oregano, crushed
- 1 tbsp red Chili powder
- 1 (15-oz.) can salt-free great Northern beans, rinsed and drained
- 1 (15-oz.) can salt-free Black Beans, rinsed and drained
- 1¼ lbs. skinless, boneless chicken breast, cubed
- 1 C. bell Pepper, seeded and chopped
- 1 tbsp Paprika
- 1 tsp ground Cumin
- 2 C. Tomatoes, chopped finely
- 2 C. low-sodium Chicken broth
- ¼ C. fresh Parsley, chopped

Directions

- In a large pan, heat oil over medium-high heat and cook the chicken, Onion and bell pepper for about 8-10 minutes, stirring frequently.

- Stir in oregano and spices and cook for about 1 minute.
- Add remaining ingredients and bring to a boil. Reduce the heat to low and simmer, covered for about 20 minutes.
- Serve hot.

DINNER

Tofu & Mushroom Curry

4 Servings

Preparation Time: 22 minutes

Ingredients

- 2 tsps Olive Oil, divided
- 2 tbsps fresh red chilies, minced
- 1 tsp ground cumin
- 3 C. fresh shiitake mushrooms, sliced
- 2 tsps arrowroot starch
- 1 tsp fresh Ginger, minced
- 2 tsps curry powder
- 16 oz. firm tofu, pressed, drained and cubed
- ½ C. water
- ¼ C. fresh Cilantro, chopped

Directions

- In a large non-stick pan, heat 1 tsp of oil over medium heat. Add Ginger, red chilies, curry powder and cumin and sauté for about 1 minute.
- Add tofu and cook for about 2-3 minutes. Transfer tofu into a bowl. In the same pan, heat the remaining oil over medium heat.

- Add mushrooms and cook for about 4-5 minutes. In a bowl, mix together water and arrowroot starch.
- Stir in cooked tofu, arrowroot starch mixture and Cilantro and cook for about 1-2 minutes or until desired thickness. Serve hot.

Tofu with Brussels sprouts

2 Servings

Preparation Time: 30 minutes

Ingredients

- 2 tbsps Olive Oil, divided
- 2 Garlic cloves, chopped
- 1/3 C. pecans, toasted and chopped
- ¼ C. fresh Cilantro, chopped
- 1 tbsp unsweetened applesauce
- 8 oz. extra-firm tofu, pressed, drained and cut into slices
- ½ lb. Brussels sprouts, trimmed and cut into wide ribbons

Directions

- In a pan, heat ½ tbsp of oil over medium heat and cook tofu for about 6-7 minutes or until browned completely, stirring occasionally.
- Add Garlic and pecans and sauté for about 1 minute. Add applesauce and cook for about 2 minutes. Stir in Cilantro and remove from heat.

- Transfer tofu into a plate and set aside. In the same pan, heat the remaining oil over medium-high heat.

- Add Brussels sprouts and cook for about 5 minutes. Divide Brussels sprouts in serving plate. Top with tofu mixture and serve.

Tofu with Spinach

3 Servings

Preparation Time: 35 minutes

Ingredients

- 2 tbsps Olive Oil
- 2 small Garlic cloves, minced
- 2 tsps fresh basil, chopped
- ½ lb. firm tofu, pressed, drained and cubed
- 1 Freshly ground Black pepper, to taste
- 1 tsp white sesame seeds, toasted
- 1 medium yellow Onion, chopped
- ½ tsp fresh Ginger, minced
- ½ tsp red pepper flakes, crushed
- 4 C. fresh spinach, chopped
- 1 tbsp fresh lemon juice

Directions

- In a medium non-stick pan, heat the oil over medium heat and sauté the Onion for about 3-4 minutes.

- Stir in the Garlic, Ginger, basil and red pepper flakes and sauté for about 1 minute. Add the tofu cubes and stir fry for about 5-6 minutes.

- Add the spinach and Black pepper and stir fry for about 3-4 minutes. Stir in the lemon juice and remove from the heat.

- Serve hot with the garnishing of the sesame seeds.

Turkey &Pumpkin Stew

5 Servings

Preparation Time: 1 hour 5minutes

Ingredients

- 2 tbsps Olive oil, divided
- 2 tsps fresh Ginger root, grated
- 1 C. homemade Pumpkin puree
- 1¼ C. Water
- ¼ C. fresh Cilantro, chopped
- 4 Scallions, chopped
- 1½ lbs. cooked Boneless turkey meat, chopped
- 2 C. Tomatoes, chopped finely
- Freshly ground Black pepper, to taste

Directions

- In a large pan, heat 1 tbsp of the oil over medium heat and sauté the scallion for about 2 minutes.
- Add the ginger and sauté for about 2 minutes. Transfer the scallion mixture into a bowl.

- In the same pan, heat the remaining oil over medium heat and cook the turkey for about 3-4 minutes. Stir in the scallion mixture and remaining ingredients except for cilantro and bring to a boil.

- Reduce the heat to low and simmer, partially covered for about 40 minutes. Stir in the cilantro and simmer for about 2 minutes.

- Remove from the heat and serve hot.

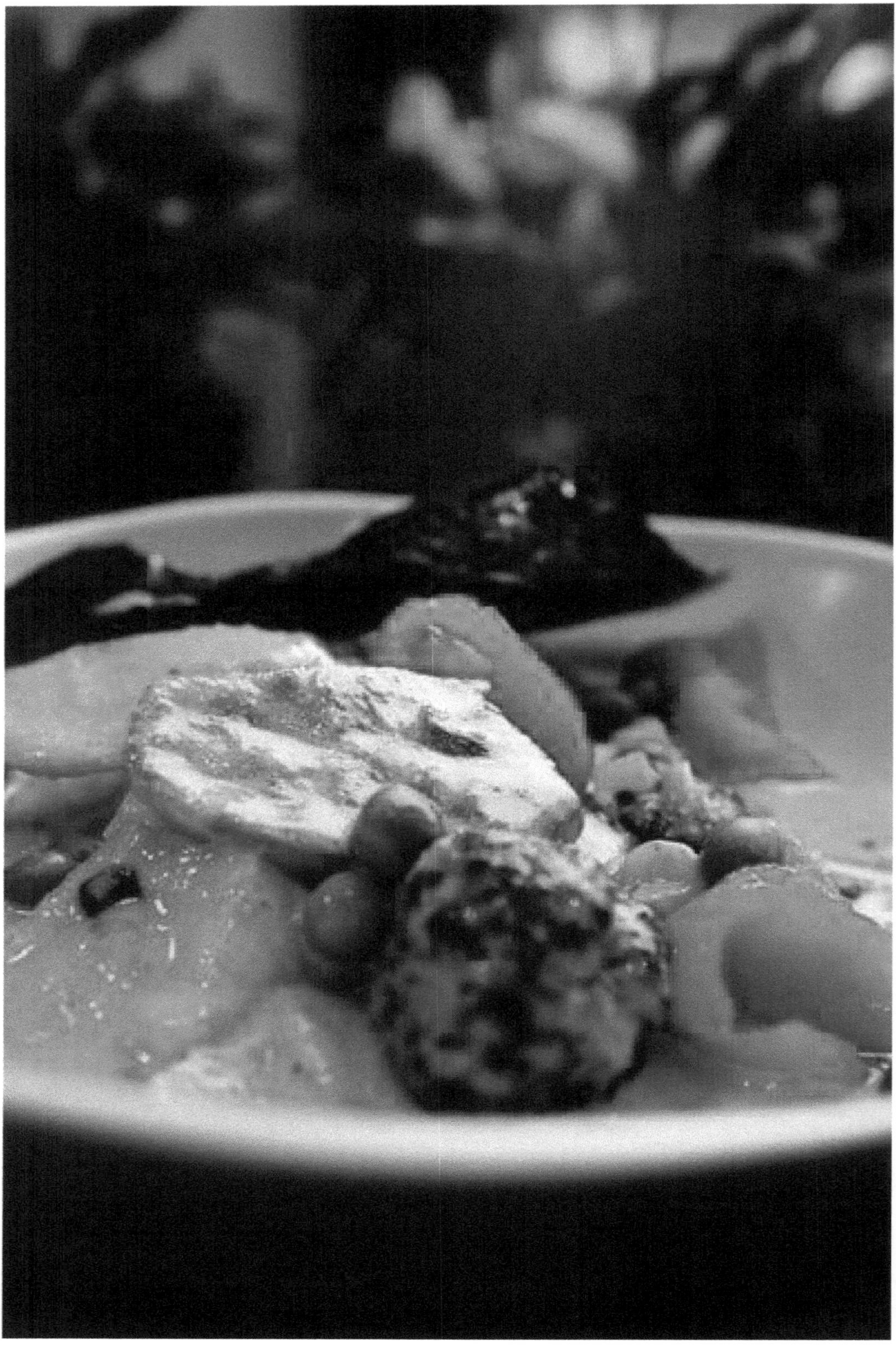

Baked Beef & Veggies Stew

7 Servings

Preparation Time: 3 hours 15minutes

Ingredients

- 1 C. Water
- 1 (2-lb.) Beef chuck roast, trimmed and cubed
- 2 C. Tomatoes, chopped
- 2 medium Onion, chopped
- 1 tbsp fresh Thyme, chopped
- 2 C. low-sodium Chicken broth
- 3 tbsps Arrowroot starch
- 1 lb. fresh Mushrooms, sliced
- 4 medium Carrots, peeled and chopped
- 2 Celery stalks, chopped
- 2 Garlic cloves, minced
- Freshly ground Black pepper, to taste

Directions

- Preheat the oven to 325 °F. In a bowl, mix together Water and arrowroot starch.

- In a large oven-proof pan, add remaining ingredients and stir to combine. Slowly add arrowroot starch mixture, stirring continuously.

- Cover the pan and bake for about 3 hours, stirring after every 30 minutes. Serve hot.

Shrimp Stew

5 Servings

Preparation Time: 35minutes

Ingredients

- 2 tbsps Olive oil
- 2 Garlic cloves, minced
- 1 tsp smoked Paprika
- 3 C. low-sodium Chicken broth
- 2 tbsps fresh Lime juice
- ½ C. Onion, chopped finely
- 1 Serrano pepper, chopped
- 4 C. fresh Tomatoes, chopped
- 2 lbs. Shrimp, peeled and deveined
- 2 tbsps fresh Basil, chopped

Directions

- In a large soup pan, heat oil over medium-high heat and sauté the Onion for about 5-6 minutes.

- Add the garlic, Serrano pepper and paprika and sauté for about 1 minute. Add the tomatoes and broth and bring to a boil.

- Reduce the heat to medium and simmer for about 5 minutes.

- Stir in the shrimp and cook for about 4-5 minutes.

- Stir in Lemon juice and basil and remove from heat. Serve hot.

Seafood Stew

7 Servings

Preparation Time: 20minutes

Ingredients

- 2 tbsps Olive oil
- 3 Garlic cloves, minced
- ¼ tsp Red pepper flakes, crushed
- 1½ C. low-sodium Fish broth
- ½ lb. Shrimp, peeled and deveined
- ¼ lb. Bay scallops
- 2 tbsps fresh Lemon juice
- 1 medium yellow Onion, chopped
- 1 Jalapeño pepper, chopped
- ½ lb. fresh Tomatoes, chopped
- 1 lb. red Snapper fillets, cubed
- ¼ lb. fresh Squid, cleaned and cut into rings
- ¼ lb. Mussels
- ½ C. fresh Parsley, chopped

Directions

- In a large soup pan, heat oil over medium heat and sauté the Onion for about 5-6 minutes.

- Add the garlic, Serrano pepper and red pepper flakes and sauté for about 1 minute. Add tomatoes and broth and bring to a gentle simmer.
- Reduce the heat to low and cook for about 10 minutes. Add the snapper and cook for about 2 minutes.
- Stir in the remaining seafood and cook for about 6-8 minutes. Stir in the Lemon juice, basil, salt and Black pepper and remove from heat. Serve hot.

Quinoa & Lentil Stew

5 Servings

Preparation Time: 45minutes

Ingredients

- 1 tbsp Olive oil
- 3 Celery stalks, chopped
- 4 Garlic cloves, minced
- ½ C. Dried quinoa, rinsed
- 1 tsp red Chili powder
- 2 C. fresh Spinach, chopped
- 3 Carrots, peeled and chopped
- 1 yellow Onion, chopped
- 4 C. Tomatoes, chopped
- 1 C. red Lentils, rinsed
- 5 C. low-sodium Vegetable broth

Directions

- In a large pan, heat the oil over medium heat and sauté the celery, Onion, and carrot for about 4-5 minutes. Add the garlic and sauté for about 1 minute.

- Add the remaining ingredients except the spinach and bring to a boil. Reduce the heat to low and simmer covered for about 20 minutes.

- Stir in spinach and simmer for about 3-4 minutes. Serve hot.

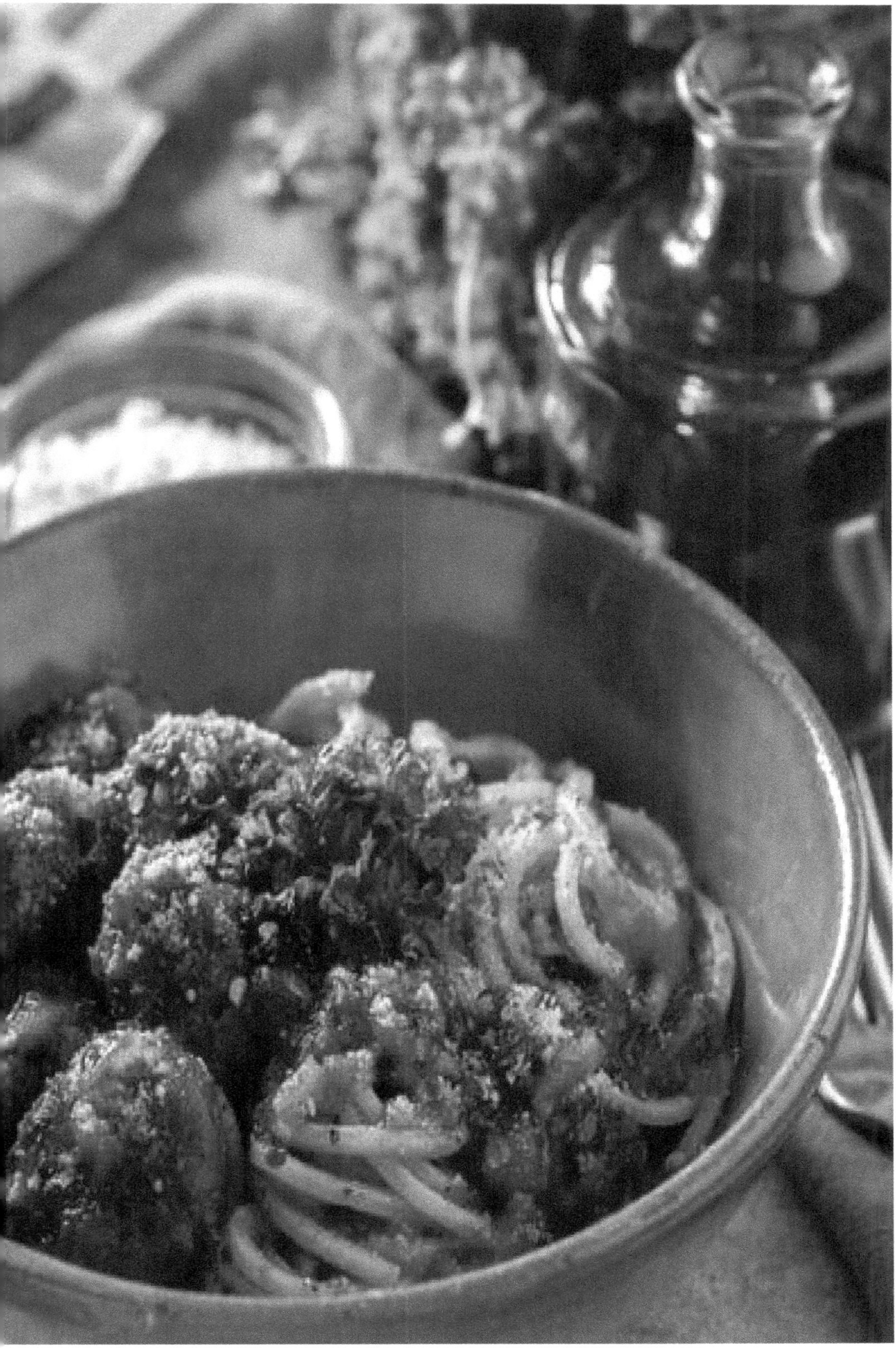

Pasta & Beans Stew

4 Servings

Preparation Time: 35minutes

Ingredients

- 1 tbsp Canola oil
- 1 medium Zucchini, chopped
- 1 tsp Garlic, chopped finely
- 1 tsp Cayenne pepper
- 2 C. Tomatoes, chopped finely
- 2 C. cooked Cannellini beans
- 2 tsps Apple cider vinegar
- 1 large Onion, chopped
- 1 bell Peppers, seeded and chopped
- 2 tbsps mixed fresh Herbs, chopped
- 2 C. low-sodium Vegetable broth
- 1 C. whole-wheat Rotini pasta
- 1 C. fresh Collard greens
- Freshly ground Black pepper, to taste

Directions

- In a large pan, heat oil over medium heat and sauté Onion, zucchini, bell peppers for about 4-5 minutes.

- Add garlic, bay leaves, herbs and cayenne pepper and sauté for about 1 minute.
- Add broth and tomato and bring to a boil. Reduce the heat to low and simmer, covered for about 15-20 minutes.
- Stir in pasta and simmer, covered for about 10-12 minutes.
- Uncover and stir in remaining ingredients and simmer for about 3-4 minutes. Serve hot.

SOUPS

Squash & Pear Soup

5 Servings

Preparation Time: 55minutes

Ingredients

- 1 tbsp Olive oil
- 2 Pears, peeled, cored and chopped
- 4 C. low-sodium Vegetable broth
- ¼ C. unsweetened Almond Milk
- 1 medium yellow Onion, chopped
- 1½ lbs. Butternut squash, peeled, seeded and chopped
- Pinch of freshly ground Black pepper

Directions

- In a large soup pan, heat the oil over medium heat and sauté Onion for about 5 minutes. Add pears, squash and broth and bring to a boil over high heat.
- Reduce the heat to medium-low and simmer, covered for about 20-25 minutes. Stir in almond Milk and cook for about 5 minutes.

- Stir in Black pepper and remove from heat. Set aside to cool slightly. Transfer the soup mixture in a blender in batches and pulse until smooth.

- Return the soup into the pan over medium heat and cook for 2-3 minutes or until heated completely. Serve hot.

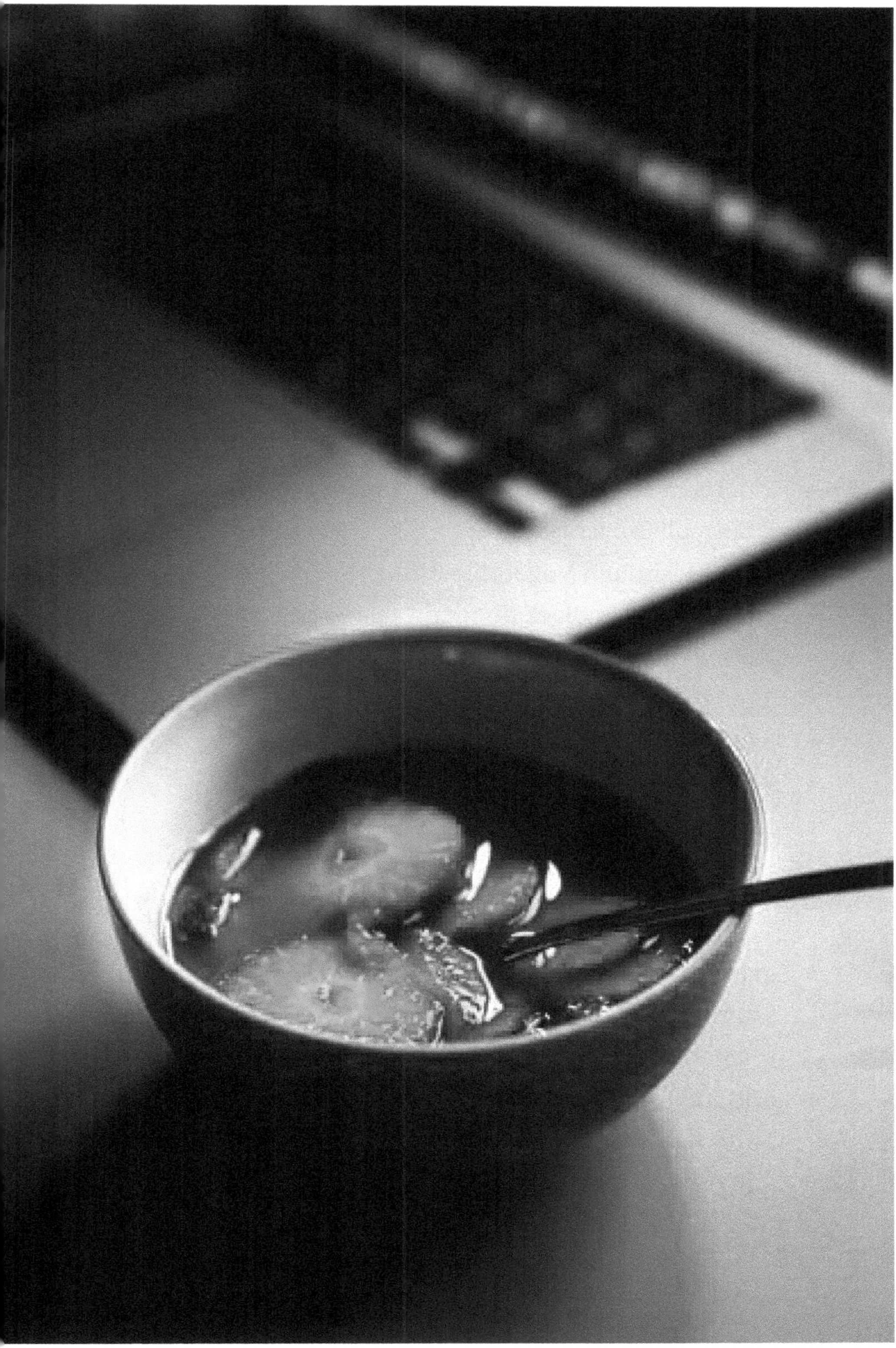

Mixed Veggie Soup

6 Servings

Preparation Time: 50minutes

Ingredients

- 1½ tbsps Olive oil
- 2 Celery stalks, chopped
- 2 C. fresh Tomatoes, chopped finely
- 3 C. small Broccoli florets
- 8 C. low-sodium Vegetable broth
- Freshly ground Black pepper, t taste
- 4 medium Carrots, peeled and chopped
- 1 medium Onion, chopped
- 3 C. small Cauliflower florets
- 3 C. frozen Peas
- 3 tbsps fresh Lemon juice

Directions

- In a large soup pan, heat the oil over medium heat and sauté the carrots, celery and Onion for 6 minutes. Stir in the garlic and sauté for about 1 minute.
- Add the tomatoes and cook for about 2-3 minutes, crushing with the back of a spoon.

- Add the vegetables and broth and bring to a boil over high heat. Reduce the heat to low and simmer, covered for about 30-35 minutes.
- Stir in the Lemon juice and Pinch of salt remove from the heat. Serve hot.

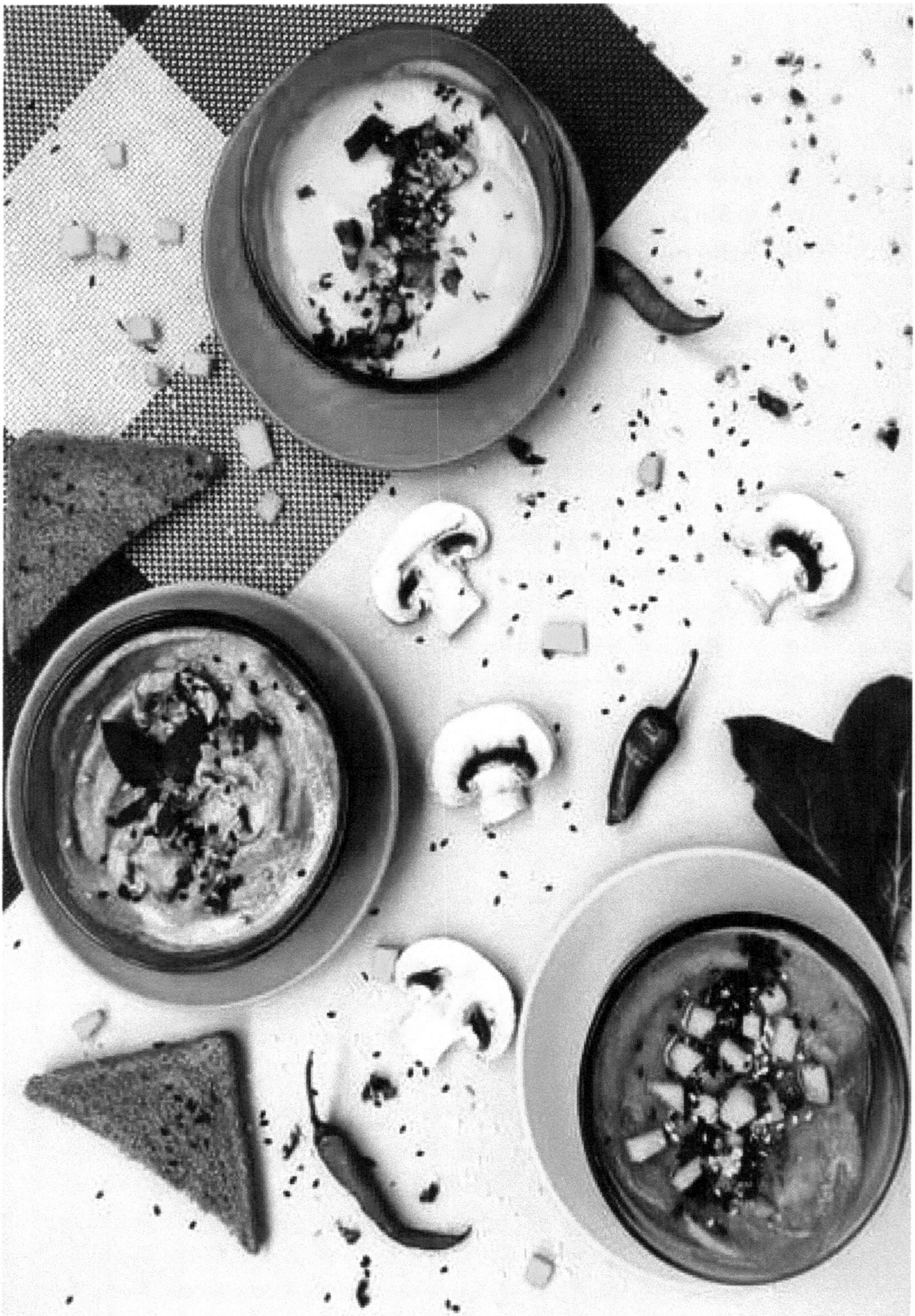

Lentil & Greens Soup

6 Servings

Preparation Time: 55minutes

Ingredients

- 1 tbsp Olive oil
- 1 medium yellow Onion, chopped
- ¼ tsp Red pepper flakes
- 1 C. red Lentils, rinsed
- 2 C. fresh Mustard greens, chopped
- Freshly ground Black pepper, to taste
- 2 Carrots, peeled and chopped
- 3 Garlic cloves, minced
- 2 C. tomatoes, chopped
- 5½ C. Water
- Pinch of Salt
- 2 tbsps fresh Lemon juice

Directions

- In a large pan, heat oil over medium heat and sauté the carrots, celery and Onion for about 5-6 minutes.
- Add the garlic and spices and sauté for about 1 minute. Add the tomatoes and cook for about 2-3 minutes. Stir in the lentils and Water and bring to a boil.

- Reduce the heat to low and simmer, covered for about 35 minutes. Stir in greens and cook for about 5 minutes. Stir in salt, Black pepper and Lemon juice and remove from the heat. Serve hot.

Barley & Chickpeas Soup

5 Servings

Preparation Time: 55minutes

Ingredients

- 1 tbsp Olive oil
- 2 Celery stalks, chopped
- 2 tbsps fresh Rosemary, chopped
- 4 C. fresh Tomatoes, chopped
- 1 C. pearl Barley
- 2 tbsps fresh Lemon juice
- 1 white Onion, chopped
- 1 large Carrot, peeled and chopped
- 2 Garlic cloves, minced
- 4 C. low-sodium Vegetable broth
- 2 C. cooked Chickpeas
- Freshly ground Black pepper, to taste

Directions

- In a large soup pan, heat the oil over medium heat and sauté the Onion, celery and carrot for about 4-5 minutes.
- Add the garlic and rosemary and sauté for about 1 minute. Add the tomatoes and cook for 3-4 minutes,

crushing with the back of a spoon. Add the barley and broth and bring to a boil.

- Reduce the heat to low and simmer, covered for about 20-25 minutes.
- Stir in the chickpeas, Lemon juice and Black pepper and simmer for about 5 minutes more. Serve hot

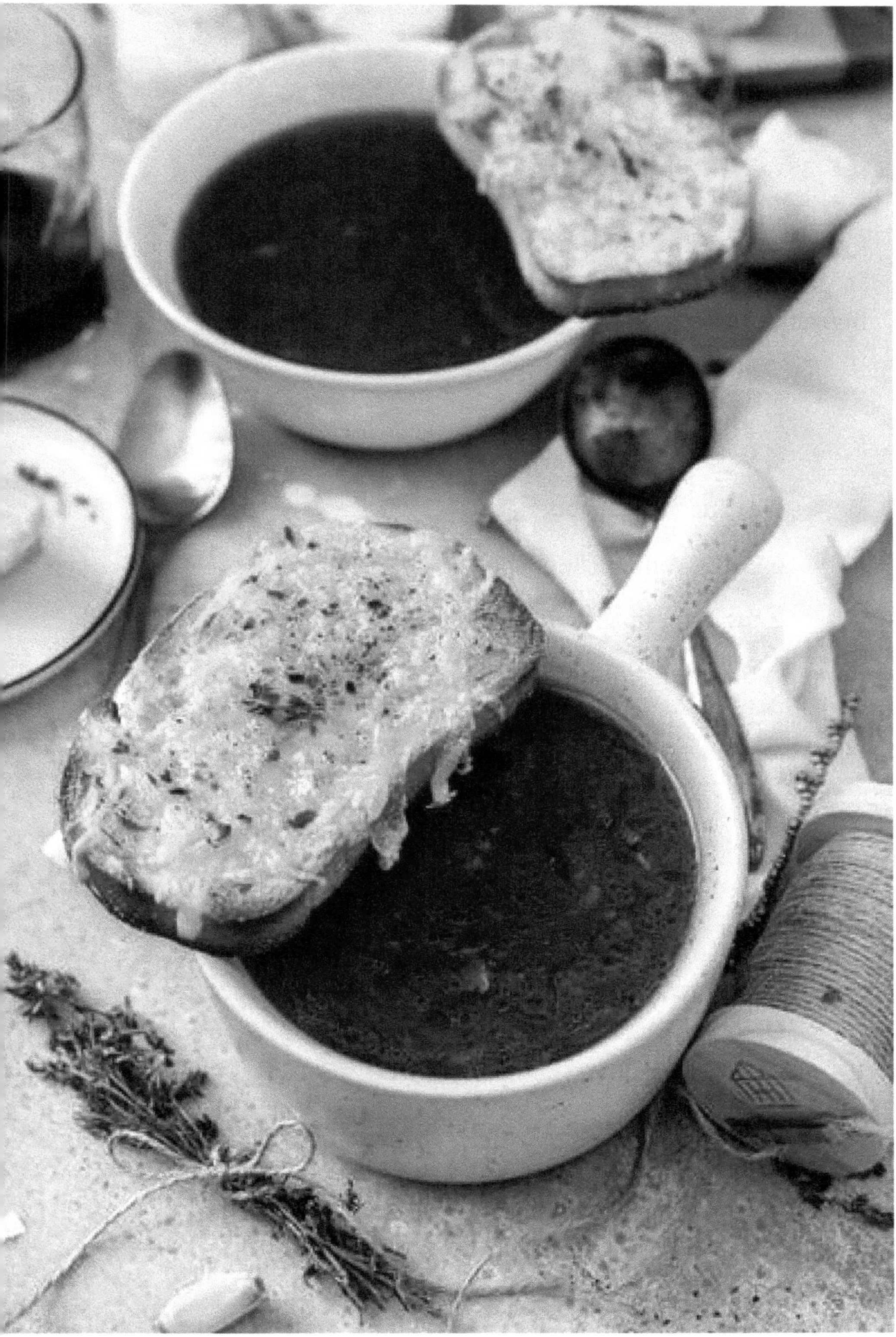

Chicken & Zucchini Soup

2 Servings

Preparation Time: 40minutes

Ingredients

- 1 tbsp Olive oil
- ½ C. Celery stalk, chopped
- 2 C. Zucchini, sliced
- 2 C. cooked Chicken, chopped
- 2 tbsps fresh Lemon juice
- ½ C. Onion, chopped
- 2 Garlic cloves, minced
- 5 C. low-sodium Chicken broth
- Freshly ground Black pepper, to taste

Directions

- In a large pan, heat oil over medium heat and sauté Onion and celery for about 8-9 minutes. Add garlic and sauté for about 1 minute.
- Add zucchini and broth and bring to a boil over high heat.

- Reduce the heat to medium-low and simmer for about 5-10 minutes. Add cooked chicken and simmer for about 5 minutes.

- Stir in Black pepper, Lemon juice and cilantro and remove from heat. Serve hot.

Beef & Mushroom Soup

5 Servings

Preparation Time: 1 hour 35minutes

Ingredients

- ¼ C. Olive oil
- ½ C. yellow Onion, chopped
- 1 tsp dried Thyme, crushed
- 2 C. Tomatoes, chopped
- 3 tbsps fresh Lemon juice
- ¼ C. fresh Parsley, chopped
- 2 lbs. Beef stew meat, cut into ½-inch chunks
- 2 Garlic cloves, minced
- 12 oz. fresh white Mushrooms, sliced
- 6 C. low-sodium Chicken broth
- Freshly ground Black pepper, to taste

Directions

- In a large pan, heat 2 tbsps of oil over medium heat and sear the beef cubes in 2 batches for about 3-4 minutes or until browned completely.
- With a slotted spoon, transfer the beef cubes into a bowl. In the same pan, heat the remaining oil over

medium heat and sauté the Onion and garlic for about 2-3 minutes.

- Add the mushrooms and cook for about 5-6 minutes, stirring occasionally.
- Stir in the cooked beef cubes and remaining ingredients except the parsley and bring to a boil. Reduce the heat to low and cook for about 1 hour.
- Stir in the Lemon juice, salt and Black pepper and remove from the heat. Serve hot with the garnishing of parsley.

Beef & Chickpeas Soup

5 Servings

Preparation Time: 1 hour 5minutes

Ingredients

- 1½ tbsps Olive oil
- 2 Garlic cloves, minced
- 3 C. Cabbage, shredded
- 1½ C. fresh Mushrooms, sliced
- 6 C. low-sodium Chicken broth
- 2 tbsps fresh Cilantro, chopped
- ¾ C. Onion, chopped
- 1 lb. lean ground Beef
- 1½ C. Bell peppers, seeded and chopped
- 1¼ C. Tomatoes, chopped
- 2 tbsps fresh Lemon juice
- Freshly ground Black pepper, to taste

Directions

- In a large soup pan, heat oil over medium heat and sauté Onion for about 3-4 minutes.
- Add garlic and sauté for about 1 minute. Add beef and cook for about 4-5 minutes. Add vegetables and cook for abbot 4-5 minutes.

- Add chickpeas and broth and bring to a boil. Reduce the heat to low and simmer, covered for about 25-30 minutes.
- Stir in Lemon juice, cilantro and Black pepper and remove from the heat. Serve hot.

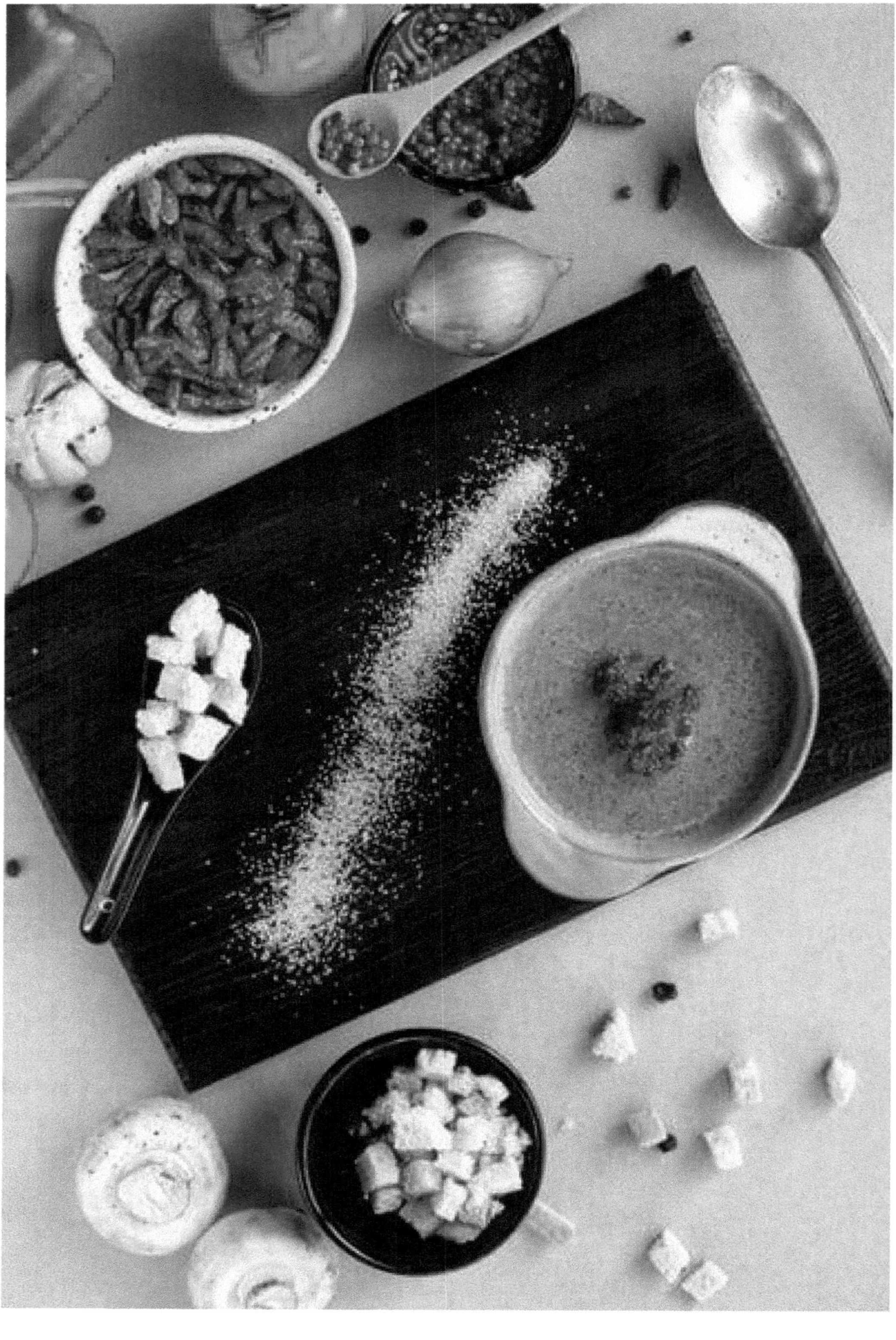

Ground Beef Soup

5 Servings

Preparation Time: 45minutes

Ingredients

- 1 tbsp Olive oil
- ½ lb. fresh Mushrooms, sliced
- 1 Garlic clove, minced
- 6 C. low-sodium Chicken broth
- Freshly ground Black pepper, to taste
- 1 lb. lean ground Beef
- 1 small yellow Onion, chopped
- 1 lb. Head bok choy, stalks and leaves separated and chopped

Direction

- In a large pan, heat oil over medium-high heat and cook the beef for about 5 minutes.
- Add the Onion, mushrooms and garlic and cook for about 5 minutes. Add the bok choy stalks and cook for about 4-5 minutes. Add broth and bring to a boil.

- Reduce the heat to low and simmer, covered for about 10 minutes. Stir in the bok choy leaves and cook for about 5 minutes.

- Stir in Black pepper and serve hot.

Salmon & Veggie Soup

4 Servings

Preparation Time: 45minutes

Ingredients

- 2 tbsps Olive oil
- 2 Garlic cloves, minced
- 1 head Chinese cabbage, chopped
- 5 C. low-sodium Vegetable broth
- ¼ C. fresh Cilantro, minced
- Freshly ground Black pepper, to taste
- 1 Shallot, chopped
- 1 Jalapeño pepper, chopped
- 2 small Bell peppers, seeded and chopped
- 2 (4-oz.) Boneless salmon fillets, cubed
- 2 tbsps fresh Lemon juice

Direction

- In a large soup pan, heat oil over medium heat and sauté shallot and garlic for about 2-3 minutes.

- Add cabbage and bell peppers and sauté for about 3-4 minutes. Add broth and bring to a boil over high heat. Reduce the heat to medium-low and simmer for about 10 minutes.

- Add salmon and cook for about 5-6 minutes. Stir in the cilantro, Lemon juice and Black pepper and cook for about 1-2 minutes. Serve hot.

DESSERTS

Vanilla Rice Pudding

6 Servings

Preparation Time: 35 minutes

Ingredients

- 1 teaspoon Cinnamon powder
- 1 tablespoon Coconut oil, melted
- 1 cup Brown rice
- 3 cups Almond milk
- ½ cup Cherries, pitted and halved
- 3 tablespoons Coconut sugar
- 1 teaspoon Vanilla extract

Directions

- In a pan, mix the oil with the rice and the other ingredients, stir, bring to a simmer, cook for 25 minutes over medium heat, divide into bowls and serve cold.

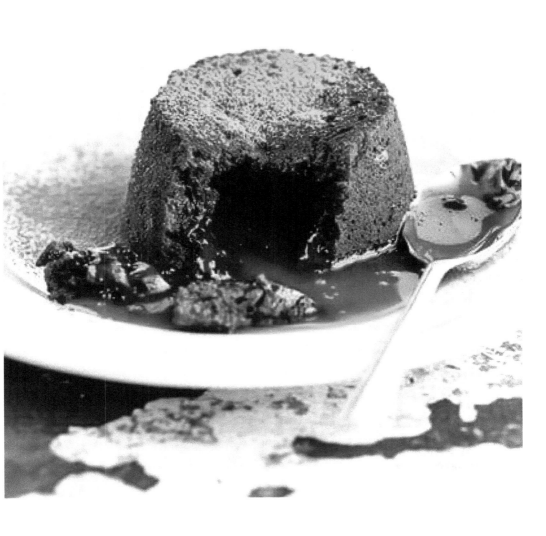

Lime Watermelon Compote

6 Servings

Preparation Time: 13 minutes

Ingredients

- 6 cups Watermelon, peeled and cut into large chunks
- Juice of 1 Lime
- 1 teaspoon Lime zest, grated
- 1 and ½ cup of Coconut sugar
- 1 and ½ cups of Water

Directions

- In a pan, mix the watermelon with the lime zest, and the other ingredients, toss, bring to a simmer over medium heat, cook for 8 minutes, divide into bowls and serve cold.

Ginger Chia Pudding

6 Servings

Preparation Time: 1 hour

Ingredients

- 1 tablespoon Ginger, grated
- 2 cups Almond milk
- ½ cup Coconut cream
- 2 tablespoons Coconut sugar
- ¼ cup Chia seeds

Directions

- In a bowl, mix the milk with the cream and the other ingredients, whisk well, divide into small cups and keep them in the fridge for 1 hour before serving.

Lemon Cashew Cream

6 Servings

Preparation Time: 2 hours

Ingredients

- tablespoons Lemon juice
- 1 cup Cashews, chopped
- 2 tablespoons Coconut oil, melted
- 1 cup Coconut cream
- 1 tablespoon Coconut sugar

Directions

- In a blender, mix the cashews with the coconut oil and the other ingredients, pulse well, divide into small cups and keep in the fridge for 2 hours before serving.

Coconut Hemp and Almond Cookies

8 Servings

Preparation Time: 30 minutes

Ingredients

- ¼ cup Coconut, shredded
- 1 cup Almonds, soaked overnight and drained
- 2 tablespoons Cocoa powder
- 1 tablespoon Coconut sugar
- ½ cup Hemp seeds
- ½ cup of Water

Directions

- In a food processor, mix the almonds with the cocoa powder and the other ingredients, pulse well, press this on a lined baking sheet, and keep in the fridge for 30 minutes, slice, and serve.

Coconut Pomegranate Bowls

6 Servings

Preparation Time: 2 hours

Ingredients

- 1 cup Pomegranate seeds
- ½ cup Coconut cream
- 1 teaspoon Vanilla extract
- 1 cup Almonds, chopped
- 1 tablespoon Coconut sugar

Directions

- In a bowl, mix the almonds with the cream and the other ingredients, toss, divide into small bowls and serve.

Ginger Berries Bowls

6 Servings

Preparation Time: 5 minutes

Ingredients

- ½ teaspoon Ginger powder
- 1 cup Blackberries
- 1 cup Blueberries
- 1 tablespoon Lime juice
- 1 cup Strawberries, halved
- 1 tablespoon Coconut sugar
- ½ teaspoon Vanilla extract

Directions

- In a bowl, mix the blackberries with the blueberries and the other ingredients, toss and serve.

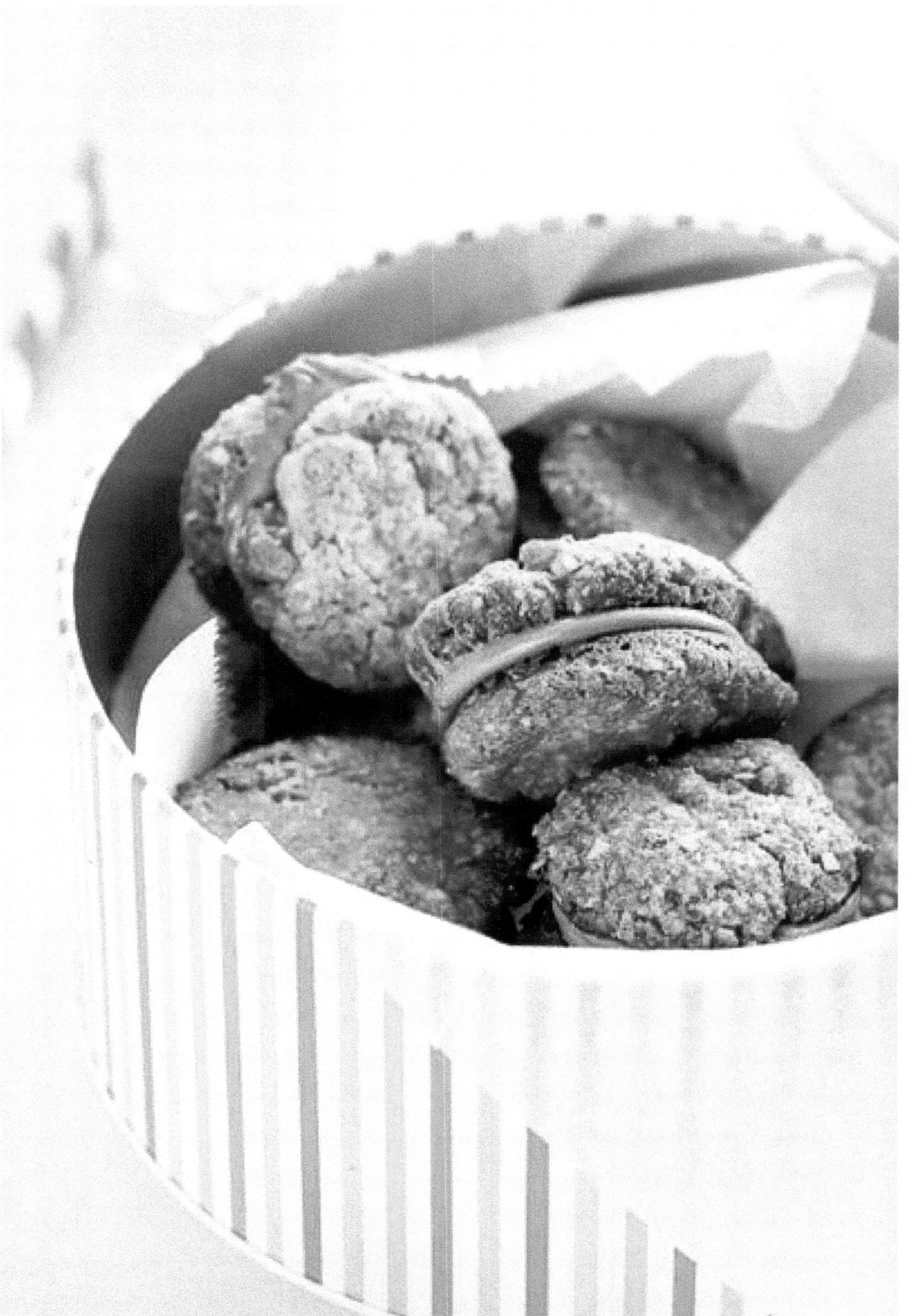

Grapefruit and Coconut Cream

6 Servings

Preparation Time: 20 minutes

Ingredients

- 1 teaspoon Vanilla extract
- 1 cup of Coconut milk
- 2 tablespoons Coconut sugar
- ½ cup Coconut cream
- 4 Grapefruits, peeled and roughly chopped

Directions

- In a pan, combine the milk with the grapefruits and the other ingredients, whisk, bring to a simmer and cook over medium heat for 10 minutes.
- Blend using an immersion blender, divide into bowls and serve cold.

Lightning Source UK Ltd.
Milton Keynes UK
UKHW020840040621
384920UK00001B/121

9 781803 005997